SWEAT YOUR PRAYERS

Also by Gabrielle Roth

Maps to Ecstasy

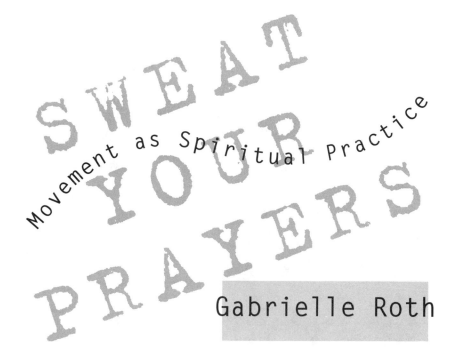

SWEAT YOUR PRAYERS

Movement as Spiritual Practice

Gabrielle Roth

Jeremy P. Tarcher | Putnam a member of Penguin Putnam Inc. | New York

Most Tarcher/Putnam books are available at special quantity discounts for bulk purchases for sales promotions, premiums, fund-raising, and educational needs. Special books or book excerpts also can be created to fit specific needs. For details, write or telephone Putnam Special Markets, 200 Madison Avenue, New York, NY 10016; (212) 951-8891.

Maude Meehan's poem "Choice," from her book *Washing the Stones* (Papier Mache Press), was used with permission, agreement dated August 4, 1997.

Jeremy P. Tarcher/Putnam
a member of
Penguin Putnam Inc.
200 Madison Avenue
New York, NY 10016

Library of Congress Cataloging-in-Publication Data

Roth, Gabrielle, date.
    Sweat your prayers: movement as spiritual practice/
by Gabrielle Roth.
        p.   cm.
    ISBN 0–87477–878–6 (alk. paper)
    1. Spiritual life.   2. Dance—Religious aspects.   I. Title.
BL625.94.R68   1998
248—dc21   97–28991   CIP

Book design by Chris Welch

Printed in the United States of America
10 9 8 7 6 5 4 3 2 1

This book is printed on acid-free paper. ∞

For my mother—
    in honor of
        her giant heart
            and gentle spirit

ACKNOWLEDGMENTS

From the depths of my heart, I wish to thank:

Robert Ansell, my beloved soulmate, the invisible force that shaped every page of this book, the brilliant presence that blesses every page of my life.

Jonathan Horan, my sweet son, for being my sidekick on the road to freedom and initiating me ever deeper into the mysteries of my life and work. I am awed by his faith and I rely on his clarity more than tongues can tell.

Kathryn Altman and Lori Saltzman, the Wicked Wits of the West, whose humor, in the best and worst of times, cracked me up, laid me low, and brought me back for more. They are my soul sisters and posse. I don't ride anywhere without them. They have covered every mile and every aspect of this journey with me. Special thanks to both of them for dropping everything but the baby to fly east so that Kathy could help me create the TO DO (or NOT TO DO) sections and for their daily injections of inspiration and feedback.

Martha Clark-Peabody, for her generous gifts of words and wisdom.

Susannah and Ya'Acov, for never being more than a fax away and their willingness to bare their souls in a heartbeat.

Christine Donovan, for catalyzing my consciousness.

Johnny Dark, for jazzlike conversations.

Terry Iacuzzo, for her wild-mind mystic mouth and downtown DNA.

Natalie Goldberg, for her zensitivity and soulful support.

Vasilisa, for her dance.

Lev Spiro, for his juicy e-mails.

Sanga, for keeping the beat.

Dr. Ming Jin, for keeping me alive.

Ruth Pontivianne and Anne Downes, for their hands, their hearts, their healing.

Lynn Franks, for being Lynn Franks.

Linda Kahn, for being my editor, savior, grammatical goddess, buddy, mentor, and midwife. Her intelligence, skill, and wisdom permeate the book.

Joel Fotinos, for being the most soulful publisher in the business as well as the coolest angel on earth. This book would not have happened without his editorial, emotional, and inspirational support.

Candace Furhman, my amazing agent, confidante, and best-dressed girlfriend, for the endless energy she gave to this project. (Jane Hogan, for turning me on to Candace.)

Irene Prokop, for her unwavering faith and intelligent guidance.

Michael Craft, for being a soulful source of inspiration.

Hal Bennett, for being a good friend, my writing coach, sounding board, and for his editorial contributions to this book.

Linda Michaels, my sweet foreign agent, for her wise suggestions and enthusiastic support.

Hans Li, for his amazing grace under pressure and tireless efforts toward creating the visual icons for this book.

Jeremy Tarcher, for his vision.

The whole Tarcher staff, most particularly Jocelyn Wright, who graciously helped me float through all the changes. Tim Meyer, for his sensitive copyediting and generous feedback.

Greg Wittrock, for digging down to the bottom of his soul and assisting us in developing the cover when he really wanted to be on the ice doing his thing.

Michelle Wetherbee, for her beautiful cover.

Pat Sweeney and Maria Duerr, for their typing.

Places where the book brewed over countless dinners at unpredictable times. I thank them for their gracious hospitality:

Gotham Bar & Grill—Laurie

Il Bagatto—Julio, Beatrice, Pilar

Indochine

Arte—Martino

Campagna

For their ferocious introspection:

Kathryn Altman, Robert Ansell, Adam Barley, Tim Booth, Martha Clark-Peabody, Jo Cobbit, Ya'Acov Darling-Kahn, Susannah Darling-Kahn, Andrea Davis, Lisa Demoney, Eleanor Devinney, Christine Donovan, Kate Engineer, Erik Larsen, Lynn Franks, Kathleena Gorga, Cora Greenhill, Jane Hogan, Jasmine Horan, Jonathan Horan, Todd Howard, Georgina Jahner, Mary Lapides, Deborah Jay-Levin, Amber Rose Kaplan, Jay Kaplan, Stefanie Kaye, Dan Lent, Jo Ann Levitt, Hans Li, Alex Mackay, Kelsey Maddox-Bell, Jaihn Makayute, Vin Marti, Nicholas Naylor-Leyland, Tierre Nirav, Zeet Peabody, Lori Saltzman, Tom Schultz, Rick Schwartz, Rick Sinderman, Clare Scott-McCarthy, Dana Shaw, Vivian Shaw, Lorca Simons, Julie Skarratt, Michael Skelton, Lori Smullin, Eliezer Sobel, Davida Taurek, Pauline Wakeham, Bruce Werner, Greg Wittrock, Maryann Wood.

Robo, our cat, for being a constant reminder of the true nature of a free spirit.

CONTENTS

Waves are the practice of the
water. To speak of waves apart from
water or water apart from waves is a
delusion. Water and waves are one.
Big mind and small mind are one.
Shunryu Suzuki, *Zen Mind,*
Beginner's Mind

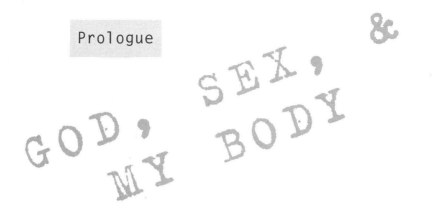

GOD, SEX, & MY BODY

F rom as far back as I can remember, I was obsessed by a gnawing hunger for rituals of spirit. When I was six I lived across the street from a fundamentalist Christian church. Every Sunday, while my sweet young parents cloistered themselves in their bedroom, I snuck out, hid in the bushes, and listened to the preacher rail against sin and the people praise God in song. I loved the singing, but I couldn't figure out why the preacher was so angry.

A strange little kid, I was mad about Jesus, mad about saints, mad about all things holy. I begged to be sent to Catholic school when I was seven. My dream came true; my parents enrolled me.

This was the same year I saw my first ballerina. I was peeking in the window of a dance school around the corner from my house when she appeared like a vision, all pink and precious and proud. I wanted to be her. For the next year, I clung to the back of a very unstable cane-backed chair struggling to learn ballet positions from a book I checked out of the library. I had only a thimbleful of talent for ballet, but that didn't stop me from dreaming.

My first dance class, mostly acrobatics, took place over a butcher shop. When I got bored I looked out the window and watched the headless chickens run around the yard doing their death dance. Eventually I got to take real ballet classes where I got a sliver in my butt and the beginnings of a severe inferiority complex. My teacher was an old woman with frizzy dyed red hair, a funny accent, and a long, thin stick. I was so worried about doing anything wrong that I did things wrong most of the time. She'd say, "Grand battement," and I'd do a grand plié. Whack! Had I paid closer attention to those chickens I would have known I had to let go of my head and follow my feet if I really wanted to dance.

In spite of the scoldings and slappings, something turned on in me when I danced, something I couldn't turn off. Something that carried me away, stretched me between two worlds, the world as I knew it and a luminous world where everything appeared dreamy and diffused, the way photographs look when the lens has been smeared with Vaseline. I never knew how long these episodes lasted, but suddenly I'd be back and I'd know that something had happened. I wasn't sure exactly what. Even though I usually felt blissed, I was afraid of being caught unaware in this magical place.

I felt this same fear in school whenever a nun would scrutinize me with her piercing eyes, eyes trained to scan for sin. One Friday, a Sister zoomed in on a piece of baloney hiding out between two slices of white bread on its way to my mouth. Big sin. Catholics didn't eat meat on Fridays, but I was so hungry I couldn't help myself. She swooped down, grabbed it right out of my mouth, and stood there staring at me, disgusted. Somewhere deep in that shapeless black habit, floating around her almost-shaven skull, I felt God trembling with a rage so big it swallowed me.

I wanted to be a saint so nobody would ever look at me like that again.

I hated my hunger, hated my body for betraying me, and in this dumb moment I swore I would never let my appetite get the best of me. Instead, I became obsessed with saints and ballerinas, emaciated untouchables. I had to get myself under control, keep my toes pointed, my stomach empty, and my mind on God. By the time I was ten my concept of self, body, sex, and sin had all been wound tightly together into a ball at the pit of my stomach. Not coincidentally, that was the year Sister Mary Alberta gave us a lecture on chastity. In a nutshell, stay a virgin or go to hell.

By thirteen I was a wreck. My body was blossoming; every day some new part of me turned on that had to be turned off. My breasts moved from triple A to double A overnight. I was scared to death of the woman emerging from deep within my bones, her irrational desires and insatiable appetites. To suppress them I took on my own black habit—coffee. Instead of eating, I drank coffee. Every day I'd deposit my lunch money in the jukebox at the cafe next to the school, playing "Earth Angel" five times in a row, imagining myself on the back of a motorcycle whizzing off to a motel with James Dean where we would devour each other with a lust bigger than the promise of a hundred heavens. Occasionally I would be snapped out of my reverie by the tantalizing smell of french fries. I never admitted to anyone, even myself, how badly I wanted to grab a greasy brown bag filled with perfectly cut fries right out of some poor unsuspecting pimple-faced kid's hands and gobble, gobble, gobble.

Instead, I prayed for the strength to withstand temptations of the flesh, to become pure spirit. I prayed to God to take my breasts back and turn my period off. I wanted to repress all that messy, uncontrollable feminine stuff, to be a good girl, get good grades, stay razor thin, angular and sharp, like Audrey Hepburn in *The Nun's Story,* which my dad took me to see at the drive-in.

Meanwhile, my parents never stopped touching each other. They were always flirting, lying together on the old green couch, retreating behind closed doors for hours on end. I yearned to be a lover too, body and soul, and I couldn't understand why, if God made my body and my body wanted sex, that could be wrong. Someone had taken sex out of God and God out of my body. I wanted to put myself back together again.

Rock n' roll became my savior. Alone in my room, with the radio blasting, I found my feet and my feet found the beat. I cranked up the music so loud it drowned out my head and all the voices telling me I couldn't, I shouldn't, I did it wrong, I wasn't good enough. I just danced.

Something inside me began to wake up. Something scary. Something huge that connected my head to my hips and my hips to my hands and my hands to my heart and my heart to my feet till I felt like I was all over the place and nowhere in particular.

In college, I fell in love with a Catholic law student. He called me "Flower." I wanted him badly and was tired of holding myself back, denying my desire. And so, one April night, we did it on a houseboat in Sausalito that belonged to one of his fraternity brothers' parents. My whole world was rocked in that boat.

The first time I made love, I got pregnant. Nothing in my life had prepared me for my boyfriend's insensitive reaction when I told him the news over the phone. I was stunned; this was the man for whom I had saved myself, battled football players in the backseats of cars, been through world wars on faded couches. So much for the fairy tale.

He called me back with a plan. Three days later, we drove across three state lines where he had arranged for an abortion. I was terrified.

Back home, I began hemorrhaging and, for about ten minutes, I figured the nuns had been right; this was my punishment. I thought I was dying, but strangely, it was easy to let go—here was my moment, my martyrdom.

And then it dawned on me—I was losing not my life but my soul. In the rush of my blood and the stream of my tears, I could feel it leaving my body. I had always thought my soul lived somewhere else, in some heavenly place waiting for me to be good enough, pure enough to claim it, but it was in me all the time. My soul was the part of me that was brokenhearted, not by some insensitive lover, but by the sacrifice of this tiny seed of a child that had awakened the spirit of mother in me.

After the abortion, I felt like a savage angel who had lost her wings and crashed to earth. It was hard to forgive myself, to forgive the boyfriend who, no doubt, had been sweating about what an unplanned child would do to his future law career. We had shared a holy moment and he hadn't respected it and that hurt. What hurt even more was that I hadn't respected it, that I had been conditioned to consider my body the enemy and sex part of the devil's work.

My prince was a toad. I had given him something sacred, something I could never take back. But I could climb out of the backseat and drive the car. Men weren't necessarily gods, I realized, even though God was cracked up to be a man. Taking responsibility for my sexual energy awakened my spiritual power, the part of me that danced past all my worldly concerns into a burning brightness that blurred all my edges and delivered me into something bigger than myself.

Throughout college, I kept dancing, and in my dance I began to forgive myself for a sin I couldn't name or remember committing, as if it belonged to somebody else but I'd gotten stuck carrying it around. It took a long time for me to trace this feeling of shame all the way back to my sister, Eve, and to understand that the seeds of my discontent were sown in her supposed transgression. This was no Bible story. The whole world was against the feminine and all I could do was dance.

I loved to work out my body but I hated the mirrors and always having to move like somebody else. One of my teachers was short with teeny little feet that did these complicated patterns about ten times faster than I could. I became so frustrated trying to cop her style. I felt as if I were ten years old again, standing at the barre, staring in the mirror, feeling like a pink elephant: ugly, awkward, and hopeless.

As awkward and hopeless as I felt, I kept showing up till an old knee injury kicked in and I was told I'd probably never dance again. I felt lost, as if I had been erased from my own dream. I'd always thought of myself as a dancer. If I couldn't dance, who was I? I slid into a deep funk. A friend of mine who was totally obsessed with her personal growth suggested I go to Esalen, birthplace of the human potential movement, and take a group therapy course.

I went but I hated it. I ended up in an encounter group in which twenty-five of us sat around in a circle and each took a turn in the middle. It was a free-for-all, a chance for the other group members to vent their "issues" about you. I came away from my turn in the center feeling completely shredded, reduced to a speck of dirt by a group of virtual strangers. I never went back. Instead, I hung out in the baths for the rest of the week and unwittingly changed the course of my life as I knew it.

There I met my first mentor, Molly Day Shackman, who ran the Esalen massage program. She probably figured she'd better rescue me from those hot sulphur baths or I'd turn into a prune, so she invited me to participate in her massage class. Two weeks later she called me in San Francisco and invited me to join the Esalen massage crew. I didn't really want to move to Big Sur, but it was time to leave the big city and try something new.

Big Sur was raw and untamed like an old cowboy movie. Every day a new Lone Ranger showed up in a rusty pickup looking for his groove. The women were on the hunt for a new kind of self, a primal, practical self, one that you couldn't find in the fashion magazines. And then there was nature. Nature ruled on this jagged coastline; storms didn't just happen, they raged, keeping us all humble, in our place. The stars were so brilliant I could wear shades at night. I had a landlord in his sixties who delivered fresh goat's milk to me wearing a pink tutu over his long underwear. He was the undisputed queen of the coast. And then there was Esalen, hub for homeless hearts and bodies that needed to be born again.

I felt liberated by the whole scene, but I missed dancing terribly; indeed, I was in mourning, sitting on the edge of a black hole feeling like a Chinese princess with bound feet. I had been cruelly cut off from a deep and beautiful part of myself, the only part that I really loved. Even though I judged it harshly, I knew this was the part of me most connected to my soul. Fritz Perls, the reigning genius at Esalen, rescued me. He discovered that I had taught movement at Agnew State Mental Hospital during college and invited me to teach movement to his therapy groups.

In the beginning I taught my classes in part of the Esalen dining room, as it was the only room with a hardwood floor. Unfortunately, one side was lined with picture windows and often during a session people would stand around outside and stare in at us. This was tragic, as the majority of my students were paralytically self-conscious when it came to moving their bodies. I was amazed by how locked up and inhibited they were, these movers and shakers. I'd put on a Stones song and try to drown out the voices in their heads saying they couldn't move. But I knew just how they felt inside those prisons of bone, having worn a chastity belt for ten years myself. I'd have them lie on their backs, then ask them to close their eyes and rock their pelvises to the beat. Most thought of my class as recess from the serious head-work they were doing elsewhere, so it was a shock when they found themselves in a sobbing heap on the floor. Sometimes two hours of moving were as powerful as two years on the couch. I discovered that the body can't lie; put it in motion and the truth kicks in.

People came from all walks of life to this mecca by the sea to confront their demons. And their demons did not want them to dance.

I was astonished to observe that, for all their Ph.D.'s and cool clothes, none of my students knew how to breathe. They weren't breathing below the neck, as if the only part of themselves they thought worthy of keeping alive was their heads. Although I could have drawn on any number of yoga exercises with strange names and postures aimed at controlling the breath, my instinct was to do the opposite. I wanted to set the breath free and release all the pent-up energies in the body that were keeping it from moving, preventing it from being inspired.

As a kid I had always been fascinated by the Holy Spirit because no one could explain it. Even the nuns stuttered and stammered over this one. Getting to the bottom of this mystery was a challenge I couldn't pass up. One day sitting in the baths it hit me: the Holy Spirit was no less than the life force, the breath itself. If I could get these people to breathe down to their toes, it would be no less than revolutionary. It seemed to me that the established order—political, religious, social, even parents and lovers—had a stake in us not reaching the depths of ourselves. Because if we were to be completely alive and spontaneous, we'd be impossible to control. My mission was clear: to seduce people back into their bodies, into their God-given power. I considered this holy work.

The more I taught, the more I realized that this was not going to be simple. Most of us were deeply afraid of the body; some people controlled every gesture they made, others abandoned themselves to food or drink or just cut themselves off and spaced out. We were big-time head-trippers, drifting far away from any real self, with no idea that there was something holy and profound happening inside of us. I'd watch people moving completely expressionless to the wildest rock n' roll song, particularly if they had a partner. Cool is cool but frozen is another thing entirely. I wanted to put my hands on their hips and melt them down. I wanted to wake them up from their collective inertia. I wanted to rattle their bones and shake their souls. And more than anything, I wanted to dance again.

It was only a matter of time before all the dances building up inside me cut loose. An eccentric crew of live drummers was part of the Esalen scene. Until I heard them I had been stuck in the three-minute vinyl groove. By contrast, these songs seemed endless.

One hot, full-moon night an irresistible rhythm struck me to the core. I couldn't resist its call. For the first time in months, I got up and started moving. I forgot my knee, I forgot everything but the beat. Under its spell, I surrendered, holding nothing back, nothing at all. Lost in the spirit of the dance I found a path, a dancing path, that took me to the deepest, most alive place I had ever been. All those years pliéing in pink toe shoes, wound up in rosary beads, addicted to jukeboxes, and doing it on an assortment of Goodwill couches, *this* is what I had been searching for.

God had spoken to me without saying a word.

My knee had healed itself. No big operations, just rest. It must have buckled under from the stress of all the heavy expectations I had placed on it. All I did was follow my energy, the way I used to do alone in my room, but this time my dad wasn't on the other side of the door yelling, "Turn that damn noise down!" The drums kept going and so did I. I danced till I disappeared inside the dance, till there was nothing left of me but the rhythm of my breath. And in the rhythm of my breath I felt totally connected, body and soul. I finally realized what holy communion was all about.

I entered another universe, shifted into a new dimension in which there were no boundaries; everything was energy and I was just a particle riding the universal wave. It was as if I were plugged in to the master current and life was charging through me, creating a clarity that I had never known before. There were seven drummers and I could hear each one of their songs and feel different parts of my body responding.

The next day it dawned on me that the revelation I'd had after my abortion was just a glimpse of what I had experienced the night before. The soul wasn't lost; it had been buried deep in our bones, driven down under by centuries of traditions designed to control our natural urges towards ecstasy. We had become alienated from ourselves as sacred beings. Now I knew what my students wanted from my work, even if they didn't know it, didn't have a word for it, or were too scared to admit it. They wanted ecstasy and I was determined to find a way to take them to that holy space.

After this I noticed a shift in my teaching, I looked at the bodies with a new eye. I became hell-bent on finding the flow of each person's energy, just as the nuns had been hell-bent on stopping mine. Where it began, where it stopped, what kind of rhythm seemed to turn it on or off. Instinct told me, you are how you move. This was the key to my emerging knowledge.

I tried to intuit the energy I had inhabited during my trance in an effort to understand this space. I wanted to know how I got in and out of this ecstatic state. I knew it had begun with my feet, then moved up into my belly and out my hands. I recalled beckoning to the drums with my hands as if pulling their vibrations into me. I had inhaled the beat and fallen into a continuum of motion with no breaks, no edges, an ancient circle, a timeless space that began and ended in my belly. I named this rhythm *flowing*.

I realized that I inhabited a different energy when I taught. It wasn't just about me anymore, but about making connections to others. I couldn't get lost in the circle of my own energy; I had to reach out and touch my students' hearts. To do this I used rock music, the pulsing 4/4 beat which contains the pain of a million puberties and gives form and shape to our longings. It was a pipeline that connected each of us to one another and to the beat of our own hearts. I began to get people to move like their heartbeat—percussive, short, sharp moves, exhaling, letting go, thrusting out. I called this rhythm *staccato*.

One night after some serious dancing, dripping with sweat and feeling totally electrified, I succumbed to a fatal attraction for a skinny white boy. This was not your wham-bam-thank-you-ma'am kind of night. He met me in my natural rhythm, my flow. Our bodies merged and he followed my movements and as the energy built, the dynamic shifted. Now I was following him, sliding into the backbeat of his heart, an irresistible drummer that swept us both away. We were one huge heartbeat that kept pumping and pumping till it propelled us over the edge into a primal pulsing space of utter surrender. I recognized this as the same place I went to when I reached the peak of my dance. My mind exploded in my body, my heart beat between my legs, and my hands groped toward God. This was *chaos*, the wild mind dancing.

I fell head over heels for this long-legged lover who wouldn't go anywhere without his dog. He listened not only to my words, but to the space between my words. He tracked my soul across my body, sensing heartaches and attitudes long buried in silent shapes that he sought with his hands to console. He kept probing, never satisfied, until he touched my most deeply-held secret, my longing for a child.

In a red brick wing of the French Hospital where I was born, just a few blocks from my old school, Star of the Sea, where a part of me had died, Dr. Kreiss told me I was pregnant. As I sat on the edge of that narrow examining table in a puke-green gown staring back at her in total amazement, I knew this was the final phase of my resurrection.

For nine months, I was in a spell. My pregnancy wasn't an easy time but the hard parts didn't touch me. I entered a state of sweet surrender, in the thrall of a force so much bigger than me I could barely comprehend it, much less control it. Instead, I just went with it, in awe at my changing body. My belly got so big I couldn't see my feet, yet I never stopped dancing. Dancing pregnant was a whole new experience. Heavy as I was, I felt translucent, like a flower hungry only for light. In this luminous space, I discovered another rhythm, the rhythm of *lyrical*. It was a state of being entranced and I knew it was deeply connected to the soul. For someone who had spent her entire life starving for spirit, what an irony to find new levels of awakening with this big belly.

My labor began fast and furious. In my natural childbirth classes they'd said I could hang around and bake cookies for a while after the contractions kicked in, but I whizzed through the *flowing* part straight into *staccato*. I still remember the walk from the house to my car because I couldn't feel my feet at all. I was a big black balloon with a strange smile on its face floating toward a Volvo, toward a whole new life. That was at 5:35 P.M. After a few hours of panting like a dog while the entire universe danced *chaos* in my belly, at 9:26 P.M. I gave a big push and out flew a seven-and-a-half-pound boy. Several doctors had predicted a girl, so for a moment I was confused by her penis. Delightenment! The *lyrical* aftermath. Totally surrendered to the forces of nature, I experienced a new lightness of being, the trance in transcendental.

The baby Buddha was placed on my breast and together we fell into *stillness*, a state that I suspect only the God within us knows. In the belly of bliss I found a new dance, one I recognized but had been avoiding since childhood, when I feared that if I sat still my world would stop and I'd fall off the edge. I was right. The world did stop, but there was no reason to be scared. I thought about how I loved that song "In the Still of the Night" back in tenth grade. I had finally made it to the still of the night and I would never again feel alone.

I went back to work with a babe on my tit and a mouth full of insights about the rhythms and how they related to life and love and sex and power and the whole creative process. Sitting in my rocking chair at 3:00 A.M., sipping peppermint tea and nursing my son, I knew I didn't know much, but I did know one thing. I didn't want my kid to grow up to hate and distrust his body, to be afraid of sex or experience it as anything less than sacred. Sex was an act of God, and I had a love baby in my arms to prove it. I had given birth to my greatest teacher. While most of my friends were running all over India in search of a guru, I'd stayed home and made up one from scratch.

Most people I knew had been taught to suppress, judge, and fear sex so that it had become a destructive force in our lives. I had gone from one extreme to the other, from being "Star of the Sea, Virgin of Virgins," to giving my body to folks I wouldn't even loan my car. The entire culture was making the same swing into a long overdue puberty. But there were consequences. A mobile V.D. clinic made a weekly visit to Esalen and the line of people waiting to be treated twisted around that funky old trailer, growing longer every week until it wound around the property and across the whole country like a tired snake. The body was talking back.

I danced through the next three decades, from disco to dharma, from Freud to Fengshui, from Kerouac to Kevorkian, from Warhol to Wayne's World, from joints to juice bars, from Gucci to the goddess to grunge, from the Beatles to the Bee Gees to the Beastie Boys. In that time I've lost scores of friends to a mean-spirited virus and seen my country go from liberal to conservative to waffling between the two. Many of my heroes have been shot down, but I'm still not paranoid. I'm faxable, feisty, and freelance and ever grateful that I missed having to deal with the second coming of condoms. I've lived to see the soul make the bestseller list and known deep in my belly the despair and yearning that put it there. Throughout it all the five rhythms have held me and rocked me, given me hope and shown me the way to bliss.

I feel my soul in my body when I dance, when I make love, and most times in between. And when I watch my students dance, I see the soul in their bodies as well. Its light, however, is most often dimmed by veils of inertia. I can't help wanting to seduce them to strip off those veils and reveal the light of their divinity. But I know that to reach the light we first have to travel into the heart of darkness. After all, isn't light created out of darkness?

I believe we each hold a spark of the original light of creation within us. I've seen it light up people's faces and bodies when they dance. In a thousand ways it has been revealed to me that God is the dance and we need only to disappear in the dance to liberate the sexual, creative, and sacred aspects of the soul.

Rhythm is our mother tongue. As I have surrendered to the wild, ecstatic embrace of the dance, I've found a language of patterns I can trust to deliver us into universal truths, truths older than time. In the rhythm of the body we can trace our holiness, roots that go all the way back to zero. States of being where all identities dissolve into an eternal flow of energy.

Energy moves in waves. Waves move in patterns. Patterns move in rhythms. A human being is just that, energy, waves, patterns, rhythms. Nothing more. Nothing less. A dance.

SWEAT YOUR PRAYERS

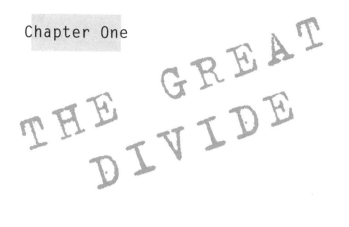

Chapter One

THE GREAT DIVIDE

To sweat is to pray, to make an offering of your innermost self. Sweat is holy water, prayer beads, pearls of liquid that release your past, anointing all your parts in a baptism by fire. Sweat burns karma, purifying body and soul.

Sweat is an ancient and universal form of self healing, whether done in the gym, the sauna, or the sweatlodge. I do it on the dance floor. The more you dance, the more you sweat. The more you sweat, the more you pray. The more you pray, the closer you come to ecstasy.

Mine is a dancing path. I have no traditions, no roots, no wise old tribal soul to give me counsel. They were burned at the stake centuries ago. Somebody got scared of shamans. Somebody got scared of people dancing till they became a sweaty prayer and fell in an ecstatic heap of bones on this Mother earth.

> I burn away; laugh; my ashes are alive!
> I die a thousand times:
> My ashes dance back—
> A thousand new faces.
>
> Rumi

After a recent workshop on a hot, muggy day, one of the participants shyly approached me and confessed that she was too embarrassed and ashamed of her sweaty body to go to lunch. I sprinkled her with China Rain, my favorite scent, and reminded her that, like a whirling dervish, she had just spent all her energy in ecstatic release and deserved a little earthly sustenance.

It saddens me that the body carries so much shame, so much fear. I guess it all started with our fall from grace, when Eve did her apple thing—I've always appreciated the fact that she offered Adam a bite; at least she wasn't selfish. So, they shared the apple and fell from spirit to flesh, and it was all her fault. And what image does the Bible throw at us to symbolize how low they have fallen, how unworthy they have become? Does it show us Adam and Eve being cruel to each other or pulling out flies' wings or burning down all the trees or eating yogurt that wasn't fat-free? No. It shows us their *naked flesh*.

And how did God make them feel? Ashamed. They fell from bliss to self-consciousness and anybody who's ever been self-conscious knows how awful that feels. What a horrible punishment—to be self-conscious about your own body, to be ashamed of it, scared of it, maybe even to hate it. A truly dismal legacy.

On a sultry summer evening in a Manhattan living room, I watched a nine-year-old Russian girl in an orange sundress with white socks doing a traditional Indian dance to a recording of a Tibetan chant. Tiny little beads of sweat formed on her luminous face. Worlds collided in her delicate hands as they floated around her body talking to God, dancing with a partner only she could see. She was Krishna one minute, Shiva the next. The whole room fell under her spell. Suddenly she stopped dancing, bowed sweetly, and blurted out, "Can I go watch TV now?"

There was no shame, no guilt, no fear hidden in her dance. She moved in and out of the divine mystery easily and unconsciously as if to her there were no mystery, as if the veil had been lifted. When Jesus said, "Enter ye as a child into the kingdom of heaven," I'm sure he didn't mean for us to imitate children but to be naked as a child. To throw down our masks and find our real face, a face that knows no shame, a fearless face. To retrieve our original innocence with no pretensions or plans, no past or future, just a fiery spirit.

This is soul retrieval, something we all need to do in order to heal an ancient and universal wound. Thousands of years ago, some men got together and, in the name of God, separated all matters having to do with the spirit from the flesh. Flesh was denigrated and the body became the enemy, its energies, passions, instincts, whims, and impulses suddenly suspect.

This was a tragic event in the history of western civilization. In this divorce of spirit from flesh, we lost respect for the body and eventually we forgot that it was part of our sacredness. In the process, we also lost respect for all things feminine, which previously had been our metaphor for all things of the earth. And, because the feminine was associated with darkness, we lost respect for the shadow side of ourselves, the part of us that lives in the deepest recesses of our psyches.

This dismemberment is our major wound. This divorce of spirit from flesh, masculine from feminine, light from dark, is the loss of

soul. The soul can only be present when body and spirit are one; it cannot breathe, exist, or move disconnected from the body. Your parents gave birth to your body, and your body is the womb of your soul. The birth of your soul is a virgin birth, one you must do on your own. It's a labor of love, and we all know labor ain't easy. If you want to give birth to your true self, you are going to have to dig deep down into that body of yours and let your soul howl.

Soul retrieval is hard work. Simply signing up for a workshop or following a guru or buying a crystal won't do it. It doesn't matter how many Buddha heads you have in your apartment if you can't find the one within you. Looking for your soul in somebody else's body or theory or fame is a lazy way to seek enlightenment. It takes discipline to be a free spirit. It saddens me that we are so quick to give our power away.

Taking up this challenge means diving into the mysterious depths of your own soul. If you aren't fascinated with yourself, no one else will be, and I've never met anybody who doesn't want to be fascinating. I'm not talking about narcissism here, but about having a dynamic relationship to the divine mystery within you—within your body, within your blood.

Think of your body as a begging bowl for spirit. When spirit is removed from the body, it is no longer inspired. And since the spirit is the catalyst that keeps all things moving, the body without it falls into a deep state of inertia. Emotions no longer move fluidly; neither do thoughts or muscles. Everything is constipated.

In this space of stuck, nothing flows together or moves in harmony. The body feels separate from the heart, the heart from the mind, and the mind from the body. Indeed, you often think one thing, feel another, and do a third, living in a state of perpetual contradiction. No wonder we're confused; no wonder we're in pain. Our soul is homeless and we can't just cross to the other side of the street and ignore it. It is the essence of who we are and to be separated from it is our deepest wound. Until we heal this primal wound and reclaim our soul, all our everyday hurts will seem big and our big hurts will feel insurmountable. The soul is the part of us that can relieve our pain by transforming our suffering into wisdom.

Pain is pain no matter what its source. Whether you have been abused or lost a limb, or had a nervous breakdown or a father who left or a mother who stayed or an addiction that swallowed you whole, the point is not your pain but your relationship to it. You can get attached to it to the point where you think it is you and allow it to define your whole life, or you can think it's special and you deserve extra points, or your self-esteem can be so low you think you deserve it. The problem is the attachment. Attachment is inertia. As with all inertia, movement of the body is the antidote.

In this book I want to focus on ways we can retrieve our souls through our bodies. Not in spite of our bodies or instead of our bodies, but through the very flesh that defines our presence on this plane of reality. We begin the process by embracing and expressing both the body and spirit, the feminine and masculine energies of our nature. In the alchemical marriage of these two forces the soul is born. It is neither and both, but a third force: the relationship between these polarities and all polarities as they exist in your nature. Your soul is a *seeker, lover,* and *artist,* shapeshifting through archetypal fields of energy, between your darkness and light, your body and spirit, your heaven and hell, until you land in the sweet moment of surrender when you, as dancer, disappear in the dance.

> *When you make the two one,*
> *and when you make the inner as the outer*
> *and the outer as the inner,*
> *and the above as the below,*
> *and when you make the male*
> *and the female into a single one,*
> *so that the male will not be male*
> *and the female not be female*
> *then shall you enter the kingdom.*
>
> *Jesus*
> *The Gospel of St. Thomas*

When your soul is in charge your life becomes a love story. And this
love story between you and yourself, between you and everybody else,
between you and the divine, is played out in specific energy fields, psychic territories that I wish to explore with you. I'd love to seduce you
into wondering about your soul; the way it moves, how it smells, feels,
tastes, speaks, acts, even what it wears. And most importantly, how it is
the part of you that makes you a fascinating, mysterious individual.

We long for our souls, for the part of us that feels moved by the rattle of Patti Smith's bones, by the raw truth of a Sam Shepard play, by
the backbeat of Jerry Garcia's heart, by the singular grace of a Joshua
tree, by the haunting shape of a Butoh body, by the cry of a lone wolf.
I lie on the floor and listen to Nusrat Fateh Ali Khan sing his "Night-
song" and I feel my longing dissolve in his. We long to be moved, to
connect with our souls.

Surfers find that connection in the ocean. Skiers on the mountain.
Monks in the chant. Actors on the stage. Drummers in the beat. I find
it in the dance.

In the beginning we all danced. Our religious roots go back at least
75,000 years to shamanic traditions grounded in the rhythms of nature:
the marvel of night turning into day, the awesome power of thunder
and lightning, the wonder of birth and death. These movements have
been our teachers and our source of inspiration, reflecting back to us
the nature of who we are. Science may have explanations, religion may
have dogmas, but the truth is we still don't know how or why the universe began to dance.

Our ancestors danced till they disappeared in the dance, till they felt
the full force of spirit unleashing their souls. This was their religion,
and it was ecstatic and personal and tribal and it moved through time
like a snake. Until it found itself in the wrong garden.

At first the church fathers were condescending. They integrated the
ecstatic tradition—hey, let them go out in the trees and do a few
dances. No problem. Who cares if they raise the Holy Spirit? The only
problem was that when the Holy Spirit actually rose, people experienced a direct pipeline to the divine mystery. The patriarchs weren't

too keen on that; it put them out of a job. People speaking in tongues, channeling the voice of God—only priests were supposed to do that. Spontaneous spiritual ecstasties were outlawed as too revolutionary, sweeping all that power back into the authority of the church. The church fathers tried to tame and control this ecstatic force, but you can't control the force of life.

The tradition of dancing into ecstasy may have been burned at the stake, but its spirit is rising from those same ashes like a Phoenix. You and I were born in the right place at the right time to once again sweat our prayers. According to Richard Tarnas in *The Passion of the Western Mind*, back in the thirteenth century there was this mystical Italian guy called Joachim who looked deep into his crystal-ball mind and saw "three eras of increasing spirituality—the Age of the Father (the Old Testament), the Age of the Son (The New Testament and the Church), and a coming Age of the Spirit, when the whole world would be suffused with the divine and the institutional Church would no longer be necessary." Could it be that we are on the threshhold of the time he envisioned so clearly? In my vision, we will dance across this threshhold.

THE LORD OF THE DANCE
I dance in the morning when the world was begun,
And I dance in the moon and the stars and the sun,
And I came down from heaven and I danced on the earth.
At Bethlehem I had my birth.

I danced for the scribe and the Pharisee,
But they would not dance and they wouldn't follow me,
I danced for the fishermen for James and John,
They came with me and the Dance went on.

I danced on the Sabbath and I cured the lame,
The holy people said it was a shame
They whipped and they striped and they hung me high
And they left me on a Cross to die.

I danced on a Friday when the sky turned black
It's hard to dance with the devil on your back
They buried my body and they thought I'd gone
But I am the dance and I still go on.

They cut me down and I leap up high
I am the life that'll never, never die
I'll live in you if you'll live in me
I am the Lord of the Dance, said he.

Shaker hymn

Mine is a dancing path. My bible is the body because the body can't lie. My master is rhythm. There is no dogma in the dance. When you let your body dance you immediately strip away the lies and the dogma until all you're left with is the spirit of life itself. Movement is medicine, and I trust that if you put the psyche in motion, it will heal itself.

There seems to be a dancing revival going on these days, from tango to tap, from samba to salsa. Not only are people longing to dance, but it seems that they're longing to dance with each other again after thirty years of dancing alone. I believe this reflects a culture-wide yearning, not only for a reunion of body and spirit, but of men and women and lovers of all persuasions. Instinct has drawn us back into the beat, back into the body to begin to sort out our confusion. Whether we turn to dances with steps, rave all night in clubs, or aerobicize till we have buns of steel, the idea is to get *moving*. Once your body surrenders to movement, your soul remembers its dance.

You have to dance through the dark in order to see the light. You have to go to the source of all our wounds, the big wound, the divorce of spirit from flesh, and heal this wound if you ever want to fulfill the longing for a real self, a soulful self, a big, huge self, one that sleeps with the Beloved.

I want to take you to a place of pure magic, where everything goes and nothing stops, like a twenty-four-hour roadside cafe with the best jukebox you can imagine. Only in this place, you don't listen to jazz, you become it. All your parts jam. It's the place athletes call the "zone," Buddhists call "satori," and ravers call "trance." I call it The Silver Desert. It's a place of pure light that holds the dark within it. It's a place of pure rhythm that holds the stillpoint. It's a place within you.

Dancing Fool

No
No monkey business
I'm not just dancing
I'm dismembering muscular memory
  and shaping the things to come
I'm not just dancing
I'm purging my media soaked soul
  of systems and Hugh Hefners
I'm not just dancing
I'm uprooting weeds that have sprouted
  in the cracks of my heart
I'm not just dancing
I'm offering my bones
  to the continental bridge
I'm not just dancing
I'm praying
I'm praying
YA, YA, SPIRIT RIPPIN' THRU
  SPIRIT RIPPIN' THRU
Rippin' thru like nobody's business
  nobody's business
  like everybody's fool
  everybody's fool
Ya, Jewel The Fool
  Jewel The Fool

Jewel Mathieson

Chapter Two

THE PRACTICE

God respects us
when we work but loves us
when we dance.

Old Sufi saying

I live in a loft building right next to one of the hottest gyms in Manhattan. I'm not a member; machines don't call me. The reality is that I demand more from my workouts—I want God. When I dance I feel the presence of a divine force and this is my addiction. Feeding it is as simple as putting on the right music and letting go. Doing what I have come to call "the five rhythms" is the surest way to drop whatever you are carrying and to move beyond your baggage to a new you, a new body, one that is fueled by its soul.

Doing the rhythms is about waking up to your most essential nature, stretching your intuition and imagination as surely as your body. It's a formless form, one that expands your range of physical and emotional expression and introduces you to forgotten parts of your psyche. It awakens intuitive intelligence and artistic sensibilities. Working out should be inspiring, not just riding some bicycle while reading *People* magazine. *People* is about somebody else, not you. Working out should be like having a conversation with your body and spirit; it should be personal, intimate, and holy, not boring and painfully repetitive.

Instead of pumping iron, I dance. Not ballet, not modern, but a different kind of dance. I've distilled the five rhythms that I discovered all those years ago into patterns of movement which I do every day as a spiritual practice, a workout for body and soul.

A spiritual practice requires consciousness, both awareness of the whole and attention to the details. As with everything else, the teaching you receive from it will be the result of the consciousness you bring to it. A spiritual practice requires discipline, the willingness and commitment to show up not just physically, but mentally and emotionally, as well. It points the way to infinity, allowing you to feel the full force of your creative genius, to make yourself up from scratch again and again. "An ounce of practice is worth a ton of theory," a wise Taoist once said.

Every morning after tea and toast, I show up in my living room in the six-by-twelve-foot space between an odd assortment of drums and an old kilim chair I bought in Santa Fe, ready to sweat my prayers. Some days I've already showered and am dressed for the street, other days I put on dance clothes. At home I always dance in bare feet.

Before I choose the music I move for a few minutes to get a reading on my energy, whether it's up, down, edgy, excited, dragging, distracted, or dreamy. Whatever I'm feeling is where I begin and what inspires my choice of music. Today I felt energetic so I chose to move to the drum workout on my *Endless Wave* CD which begins with a Rumi quote: "Dance until you shatter yourself," a reminder of why I dance— not to look pretty or perfect a series of steps, but to surrender myself to the spirit of movement.

As I move through my body, beginning with my head and ending with my feet, I consciously offer each part of myself to the dance. First I isolate the part, moving only my head, for example, and then I get behind it with the rest of my body, allowing my head to lead my body. I do this with an attitude of prayer, surrendering myself to the dance and letting it guide me through inner landscapes of bone and blood, of heart and hands, of dreams and desires.

I listen to each part of me, sense its energy, allow its story to unfold. My head, with all its preconceived ideas, beliefs, and dogmas, controlled my hips for two thousand years and now they are making up for lost time. Today they want to shake and do huge circular moves. My right hand is still holding on to some old anger I can't quite reach. I clench it in the beat but it tells me nothing new. Today my knees are wimpy whiners, but my elbows are raven's wings. My spine feels loose and snaky and a crick in my neck is trying to tell me something. All I do is keep my mind open and pay attention, letting my body parts speak to me through movement, acknowledging and releasing their comments and complaints, moving toward that inspired state of being where there is nothing left of me but my soul.

The music changes and I am in *flowing,* the first rhythm. I break out of my six-by-twelve space and follow my feet up and down the narrow hall past my kitchen to the bedroom where I wave to the beaded silver wolf robe and the golden Buddha head from Bali hanging on the wall. I curve around and go back down the hall, pulling my attention into my belly each time I inhale and releasing my body to make all kinds of circular moves. Today I am really in this rhythm, digging the fluidity. I move like blood, heavy and round. Before I have a chance to become bored the music changes.

Like it or not, I am in *staccato.* Today I like it. My body contracts, forcing me to exhale sharply from deep in my belly. The strength of the exhale thrusts out my arms in sharp, angular bursts. I punctuate space with my presence, doing the dance of my bones. I feel real funky and powerful, as if I could tackle anything—even clean my office. I empty my head into my exhale and let both brain and breath go. The cat stares at me from the couch. He doesn't get this rhythm. Little does he know, I've learned a lot about *staccato* from watching him, the way he sometimes moves like Bruce Lee on Quaaludes. I blow the cat a kiss and pretend I'm Janet Jackson. The music changes to *chaos* just as I'm lamenting the fact that I don't have her hair or her butt, and that I can't move like her brother, the undisputed lightweight champion of *staccato.*

I can't think and do *chaos* at the same time, it's one or the other, so I shake all thoughts out of my head and give all my attention to my feet. They shift my weight from left to right, releasing my back, my shoulders, my elbows. The djembe beat pulses through my body, rocking me in a riff that won't let go. I feel trippy and tribal as a wash of joy spreads over me. Suddenly my head pops back, reminding me of all the things I have to do today, and I get really distracted, moving in and out of the beat as I move in and out of my head. I struggle to let everything go and just keep dancing. I pause for a drink of water and then drop back into the beat. Just as I let go of another layer, the beat shifts.

In *lyrical,* the drums are as incessant as in *chaos,* but they have a lighter tone. I dance on my toes, basically the same movements I was doing before but with a different intention. As I skip past my plants, the ficus winks at me. Plants live in the *lyrical* rhythm, bending their will toward the light. I imagine myself a tiger lily and feel my culture, my conditioning, and all my mundane concerns fall away. The beat sweeps me into another dimension, one in which I feel flooded with light, as if I had a rainbow inside me. My feet are as light as a feather, my heart is on fire, my head is empty.

In this state of grace I slip into the rhythm of *stillness,* into the breath of the beat, to revolve around my own axis, to shift down into the drift of a waking dream. I become a series of dissolving shapes. The details of my apartment fade into the bright white light that floods in through the floor-to-ceiling windows. My body feels empty, a cavernous space supported only by a scaffold of bones. I am surrounded by empty space, inside and out. I feel an electric attraction, as if to a lover. This is my Beloved, this invisible force that makes me dance, that moves in and out of me without a trace. In the circle of my breath, I reach the stillpoint inside the dance. Moving in slow motion, I sense the vastness in every second. Borders shift and disappear; there is no inner, no outer. I seem to be everywhere.

The phone rings. The machine picks up and I can hear the voice; it seems light years removed. I hear it but do nothing about it, not even think.

Today I danced for thirty-three minutes and made it through all five rhythms. Yesterday I danced for fifteen minutes, tomorrow I may only dance for five. The Wave, as I call it, is a flexible practice, meant to reflect the level of your energy rather than force you to conform to it as a rigid discipline. The only discipline it requires is for you to show up and be true to the part of yourself that is committed to moving. Although there are five rhythms, today you may only do one and tomorrow you may do three. There is no "right" or "wrong" way to do it. You'll soon learn to listen to your body and to do what's appropriate for you in the moment. We're constantly changing and any practice meant to serve our authenticity should reflect our fluid nature.

A practice should never become routine, something you do by rote, unconsciously, mindlessly. In the early years at Esalen I gave massages in the exact order that Molly Day wanted them done. One day during lunch, the image of a long, hairy leg kept popping into my head and finally I realized it belonged to the man I had massaged that morning. It dawned on me that I had not massaged the front of his left leg. I was so into the routine of my massage that while my hands were kneading his body, my head was making a grocery list. That was the last by-the-book massage I gave. From that day forward I listened to the body I was touching and let my hands follow my impulses and intuitions. I concentrated not on the technique, but on just staying present, in the moment, mindful. Years later, at Marine World in Florida, I begged the marine biologist to allow me to watch when he worked with the dolphins. He said fine, but added, "We never know when they are going to show up. We follow their moods. If we made training into a routine, they would simply stop relating to us." I do my practice in the spirit of the dolphin and I invite you to do the same.

As to how often you should do it, I offer you another story. In the early seventies I was living in Los Angeles and studying tai chi with an amazing master. The only problem was that his class took place in a park at sunrise. Being a night person, I found this a major challenge, and I didn't always live up to it. I showed up every other day or so, but my friends went every day religiously and looked down on me because of my lack of commitment. Finally I felt so guilty I went to the teacher after class one morning and stammered, "You are an amazing teacher and I really do love tai chi, please don't take my laziness personally." He smiled an inscrutable smile and said, "No worry. One day come, one day no come, perfect tai chi," giving me permission to do it in my own rhythm.

Excuses, Excuses

In the months before I was graduated from college, I asked all my friends about any and all excuses that they had used to get out of class when they were in high school. I'd just been hired to teach English, drama, and history to tenth, eleventh, and twelfth graders. I collected about 120 excuses—I had creative friends. I mimeographed this astounding compilation and passed it out on the first day of school to all my students saying, "If you can think of anything that's not on my list, please, be my guest." I felt a little bit sorry for the other teachers, but a girl's got to do what a girl's got to do.

I mention this because you can probably think of 120 excuses why you can't or won't dance. I've heard them all and I'm not impressed. Here are my top ten:

1. I hate my body.
My friend Lori is a feisty, curly-haired queen of the racquetball court who drives fast, cracks her gum, and loves camping. She's a corporate consultant and part-time Outward Bound instructor, the kind who climbs trees and leaps off cliffs. Over a latte one rainy December day

shortly after her fortieth birthday, Lori told me an amazing story. On the last day before her thirtieth birthday, she went alone to the top of Mt. Tamalpais in Mill Valley to watch the sun set on her twenties. Sitting there she got really sad thinking about how she had spent the past ten years desperately trying to lose the same ten pounds. On the night before her fortieth birthday, she returned to the top of Mt. Tam to watch the sun set on her thirties. Yet again she mourned all the time and energy she had spent hating her body over those same ten pounds—twenty years of living in the shadow of the scale. "I step on the scale to see if I am a worthwhile person each day. I even dry my hair before I weigh myself, just like my mother used to." It turns out her mother has been battling these same ten pounds all her life, too.

"Those ten pounds are probably the most important part of you," I told her. "Think of them as a family heirloom, passed from generation to generation. Relish them. They're no different from the other hundred and twenty pounds of you except for your attitude about them. It's not like you're a serious couch potato. If those pounds haven't been scared off of you with all your daredevil leaps and climbs, if they haven't evaporated along with all those pearls of sweat you've released in the rhythms, they are meant to be part of you. Not everybody's meant to be a waif with pancake tits and hips like an adolescent boy. You are made in your own image and you are divine."

While warming up in a recent class, we got to hips and I said, "Use them, folks, the more you have the better." There was an audible gasp of delight in the room. It made me think of my friend Myrtle who has spent the last forty or so years desperately desiring smaller hips. I keep telling her, "Check your bones, it ain't gonna happen." She attended one of my theater workshops several years ago where, during a performance piece on the body, a beautiful black woman stood on stage, hands on ample hips, and looked the audience straight in the eye. "These are my hips," she announced with a sensuous swivel. "I seduced my man with these hips, made love with these hips, carried my babies with these hips. I *love* my big, black hips." I looked over at Myrtle—her mouth was hanging open. "Eat *that* attitude up!"

2. I don't dance.

Iris, a sweet, docile, though tightly-wound woman in her early thirties, came to a *Waves* workshop with a friend of hers who had convinced her it would help her to relax. She tried to talk her husband into taking the workshop with her. "You may dance, but I don't dance," he said. "I don't need to. I don't want to. I don't like to dance. Dancing is for wusses, not for people who make their way in the world by their wits." This guy had major attitude.

Toward the end of the workshop I looked up and saw this tall, angular man with piercing gray eyes speaking to Iris. It was her husband, who had arrived an hour early to pick her up. After a few minutes of persuasion, she convinced him to wait in the room.

We were in this funky downtown space and the drummers had fallen into one of those zones where they were perfectly connected to each other and to the dancers. The energy was flowing back and forth in a pulsing trance. Even the floor was shaking. Out of the corner of my eye, I caught Iris's husband tapping to the beat. I don't think he even knew it was happening; his knees relaxed and he started to keep time with his hand. He forgot that he didn't dance.

A few weeks later, I heard from Iris. She called to thank me for the teachings and to let me know that on the last night of the workshop, she had seduced her husband with a newfound passion. The rhythms rocked their bed. The next day he'd asked her, "When are you going to take one of those dance workshops again?"

3. It's too late, I'm too old.

I first noticed Evelyn, a woman in her mid-sixties, because she was huddled in the back corner of the room in one of my summer workshops at Esalen. She looked like a silver origami bird, wings all folded in on herself. I saw the fear in her eyes and wondered how on earth she had ended up in this workshop. Indeed, this particular class was filled with hot, hormonal, hip, high-energy singles and it was pumping.

After the session I went over and sat down with her to see how she was doing. She told me she had grown up in a fundamentalist household where dancing was not allowed. She had two children and three grandchildren and was entertaining the concept of retirement after twenty-five years of teaching nursing. "It's time for me to move," she said with a twinkle in her blue eyes. "But, I may have bitten off more than I can chew." She had signed up not only for the weekend, but also for the following five-day program. Her arthritis was acting up and she was looking for a way out. I told her to do what she could do and when she wasn't dancing to watch and listen. She ended up hanging in there for the full five days, dancing herself right into a new frame of mind.

After the workshop she cut back on her arthritis medicine and began to do the rhythms regularly at home. She's been moving ever since, not only physically (she's dropped a lot of weight), but emotionally, as well. Last time I saw her, she was wearing a flowing silk skirt and bright red nail polish. She's joined a tribe of dancers who all adore her and treasure her as an inspiration, an elder, a wise woman. She plugs into their energy and uses it to spark her own. She goes to class twice a week and has begun to teach other seniors the five rhythms. It's never too late to find your flow.

4. I don't have time.
A student of mine who is an emergency room doctor works sixteen-hour shifts. In between patients and traumas, he can be found in his office, door shut, Walkman on, shoes off, dissipating the tensions of his job in a dance of release. It only takes a few minutes to transform your world.

5. I have no sense of rhythm.
Reality check. You are rhythm. Ask any nuclear physicist and she will tell you that the whole universe is in constant motion and you are probably not the exception to the rule.

You breathe. You walk. You eat. You make love. You do this all in rhythm. Even when you say, "I have no rhythm," there is rhythm in your delivery.

So, since movement is the nature of the universe and you're in it, I suggest you move.

6. I am too depressed to move.

Depression is stuck energy, sadness that hasn't been released. The only way to get over your depression is to move. Ya' Acov, a dear student and friend of mine, called to tell me that after leading a long intense workshop, he came home just as his phone began ringing. It was a hospice nurse calling to tell him his best friend had died that afternoon after a long battle with AIDS. He went straight into his dance room, lit a candle, closed the door, put music on, and danced through his ripping grief, his anger that his friend had left. "I put the music on real loud and began to shout to Neil all the memories he left behind and all the teachings. I thought, 'Why wait for a funeral?' Light a candle and send him all my crazy dances. I thought about his dancing and how no beat could hold it, how he danced a thousand rhythms and all of them with a *lyrical* flair. I cried and danced and cried and danced myself through wave after wave. I spoke to my friend, prayed for his safe passage, and thanked him for his friendship. In the *stillness* I imagined myself kissing his unshaven cheek, tasting his tears. My practice comforted me and helped me to let him go."

It's in moments of crisis that we realize why we spend hours each week in spiritual practice. When the floor falls out from under you, it's your safety net.

7. I don't have a lot of energy.

My friend is a writer and wants to save all her energy for writing. She sits zazen to still her mind. I say to her, the fastest way to still your mind is to move your body. It works for me every time. The deeper I dance, the more energy I have, because I release all the stuff that's blocking my flow. All that inertia just turns into negative thinking anyway. It takes a lot more energy to repress movement than it does to surrender to it. Now *that's* exhausting.

8. I've got more important problems to deal with.

Occasionally I hit a wall, come up against a problem for which I can find no solution. It always helps me to focus on the issue for a few minutes and then drop it in the dance. It seems everybody has been coming to me with their problems recently. "Should I renew my lease?" "Should I move in with my boyfriend?" "Should I cash in my stocks?" "Should I cut my hair or go to Spain?" My prescription is always the same. Just dance for thirty minutes or however long it takes to release the problem from your mind. After a hard dance, when your heart is pumping and your breath is struggling to move deeper into your body, when you've achieved a state of energetic emptiness, the answer you've been searching for often just pops up.

9. I don't have the space to dance.

Okay, so you have a roommate who hates music, can't stand dancing, and would only judge and ridicule you if you were to break out in an amazing series of moves that would dazzle anyone else. Or you live in an apartment smaller than your average closet. You may not be able to move or get rid of the roommate, but you do have other options.

Pick the kind of music that turns you on and find a club that features this music. Go alone and dance alone—for yourself, by yourself, in spite of yourself. That way you won't be worrying about anyone else—pleasing them, showing off for them, or even worse, critically comparing yourself to them. When I was young and high-wired and needed a place to dance until there was nothing left of me, I used to go to gay clubs. They played the hottest music and nobody interrupted my dancing to hit on me—what a relief!

I have acting students who do the rhythms in an odd assortment of bathroom cubicles all over Manhattan to prepare for their auditions. A lawyer I know uses the bathroom outside his office for little dance-breaks throughout the day. I've spent half my life in hotel rooms, dancing in the narrow space between the bed and the TV.

10. I'm shy and self-conscious. I could never dance in front of people.

Self-consciousness can reside in your head or your body. I have a student who is terminally shy except when he dances. When the music comes on, he's Mr. Confidence, thrusting his body forth, asserting his right to be, releasing his most brazen self. He takes refuge in the dance because it's the only place where he doesn't feel intimidated or at a loss for words. He doesn't care who's watching until he stops dancing and the veil descends again.

Another student is a motor-mouth, a social chameleon who can be whoever she wants to be—as long as she is in her head. She can dazzle with you with Shakespearian quotes, oddball references to obscure biological facts, but as soon as we begin to move, she looks like a lone teenager cruising a strip mall in the twilight zone. She does not live in her body and is acutely sensitive to how uncomfortable being in it feels.

Self-consciousness absorbs the life force faster than a sponge. There is no way out but through it. When it hits me, I exaggerate it and turn it into a character dance, as if I were an actress playing somebody else. I've gained some perspective on my self-consciousness and learned that the most effective weapon against it is a sense of humor. Self-consciousness doesn't move; it's like being stuck in the groove of a record. The irony is that in this state of consciousness we think everyone is watching us; the truth is, this kind of behavior doesn't catch anyone's attention but your own.

Here are my runner-ups.

1. *I need steps so I can tell if I'm doing it right.*
   There is no right.
2. *Been there. Done that.*
   Confucius says: "He who departs from innocence, what does he come to?"
3. *I have this little fever and my back kind of hurts and I think I have that fatigue thing—what's it called? Do I look okay to you?*
   You look okay but you sound pathetic. You really need to dance.
4. *Show me the floor, I can outdance anyone.*
   Self-importance is most unattractive and dull. I'm yawning.
5. *If only I had taken dance classes when I was a kid.*
   That was then, this is now.

6. *I prefer to watch others dance.*

We dancers are fascinating, aren't we?

7. *What kind of dance? Where? How will I know what to do? When is it? What should I wear? Who will be there? Oh my God, I don't know if I can do it.*

Put all this energy into a panic dance. It'll be brilliant.

8. *Great! I'll splurge on one of those nifty French leotards. And, of course, I'll have to go by Tower Records and pick up some new sounds. Before I start I need new speakers. I think I should build a dance space onto the back of the house. Maybe I'll even take the teacher training. When did you say the class was? Tuesday. Oh, I have tennis on Tuesdays.*

How's the weather out there in the future?

9. *I need a few stiff drinks before I can dance.*

Perrier or Poland Spring?

10. *Not in this lifetime. Not in this body. Pass me another donut.*

Focus on the hole.

The Only Dance Lesson You'll Ever Need

> . . . *anchored in the old straight*
> *tracks of me*
> *arms wingspun in dance*
> *break with the postures of*
> *apology.*
>
> Cora Greenhill

So, how do you "do" the rhythms?

Only you can answer that. Every day you choose your own way to do the rhythms because what you need changes from day to day. Some days it's better not to move at all. Today you may need to move deep and slow but not long; tomorrow you may need to energize yourself with a wild, *chaotic* dance.

Ideally, you do the rhythms every day. But sometimes you just have ten minutes. Other times you have no minutes, so do it on the way to the subway or in the parking garage or in the elevator on the way up to your office. Sometimes your kids won't give you a moment to yourself, so seduce them into doing it with you. Sometimes you have no access to music; use this as an opportunity to follow your internal beat. Sometimes the phone rings in the middle of your practice and it's someone you must talk to or die. Pick up the receiver and keep dancing—cordless comes in handy. Sometimes you just can't get out of bed, so invite a lover over, put on some sexy music, and do the five rhythms like only you can!

Everyone has to find their own way. Some do it every day at the same time like clockwork—they jump out of bed and start dancing. Other people do it more randomly, less often, or differently every time. It's a flexible practice, one that can be done anywhere. Often after dinner at a restaurant, my sweetheart and I walk home, sometimes covering fifty city blocks without even realizing it. I take this opportunity to feel the rhythm inside my walk: in the winter I move in fast *flow* with a big stride and in the summer my gait slows way down. And then there's my man—I speed up for him, he slows down for me. While I wait for him to stop at Häagen Dazs for a coffee chip, I stand on the corner watching the *stillness* of my breath, the *chaos* of the traffic, the distinctive dance of each passerby. Life is rhythm.

"Doing the rhythms" is just applying your awareness and attention to the energies you already inhabit. Movement practice gets all your creative juices flowing. It doesn't just release your body, but it opens up your heart and empties out your mind, as well. Whatever you are feeling or obsessing over is integrated into your dance. You move away from your surface and get in touch with a deeper, wiser you, one that senses the unity that underlies everything. The rhythms take us back to that primordial soup, so that we can begin again, fresh and fertile, high on our own existence.

To help you prepare for doing the rhythms, here are five concepts to consider.

1. Destination/Direction

The goal of movement practice isn't just to get the rhythms done so you can cross them off your list. It's to do them for the sake of doing them. We've become so destination oriented that we've lost our sense of direction, our ability to follow our own instincts, signals, and inner messages. Somehow it's become more important to get wherever we're going than it is to enjoy the scenery along the way.

I learned this from eight Thorazine-whacked patients at a psychiatric foundation in the Midwest. Every day for two weeks they came to me for movement therapy. Their eyes were lifeless as they shuffled into the room; they didn't seem to have even a gesture left inside them. They broke my heart. I had no idea what to do with them—just the anticipation of them coming through the door was enough to wipe me clean of cleverness. They were so far away from any kind of self, reaching them seemed impossible.

I'd beckon them toward me with my finger and my most seductive radio-inspired voice. They'd wobble in my direction and once they got real close I'd say, "Okay, beautiful, now back up." They would trudge backward until I asked them to stop and move sideways, first to one side, then to the other. And then the high point, "Now just turn around in place." On the fifth day, a furtive-looking young man with furrowed eyebrows and hair that stood on end actually smiled while doing this. I read this as a sign of success.

Every day we did this routine, and every day they responded a bit more, until toward the end of my second week I actually got them to do this walking meditation to the beat of a popular song. In the last session, something broke through and awakened a sense of direction in them. They began deciding for themselves whether they wanted to move forward or back or sidestep or circle around. I was so happy, I wanted to roll all over the floor and cry.

When I got back to Esalen, I turned this experience into a walking meditation that I did with all my groups. I would demonstrate the five directions, and then ask them to move through the room seeking the empty space, letting the emptiness dictate their journey. Depending on the level of surrender in the room, I would speed up the tempo, increasing the risk and, if I was lucky, the consciousness. Too often, however, people just "did" the exercise, forcing their way through space with specific destinations in mind: "Now I'll do the periphery. Now I'll go to the center. I'll beat him to that space." Having no destination or being destination-driven are two sides of the same directionless coin.

When I was a kid I hated huge strangers hanging around my magical world with phony smiles asking stupid questions like, "What are you going to be when you grow up? A nurse? A movie star? A veterinarian?" I always felt as if I were supposed to know something I didn't know or be something I wasn't. From an early age we're conditioned to set goals and look toward the future rather than to pause and reflect on the present. We become so destination-oriented that we lose our native sense of direction, that inner sense of who we are and where our individual impulses and desires are taking us. This walking meditation became a metaphor for life. Sometimes in life it's necessary to move straight ahead; other times it's better to back off or sidestep or move around in the same circle until you sense a way out.

Sometimes I think those eight patients were Zen masters in disguise. They taught me how to slow down and get really simple, and that's the first thing we have to do in this practice. Follow your impulses, whims, and attractions; let them lead you off the beaten track. You don't have to rush straight through from *flowing* to *stillness*. Maybe today you won't get past *flowing*. Or maybe you'll begin and end in *chaos*. This practice is meant to realign you with instincts that have been buried deep in your bones. Learn to trust them and you'll never have a bad trip.

To Do (or Not To Do)

Destination/Direction

When I was in college I spent weekends in San Francisco with my boyfriend who was studying law. Every Monday morning I walked with him to school, and to my astonishment he always took exactly the same route. I was way too curious an individual to ever do things that way. I wanted to explore and get to know the whole neighborhood.

This week when you go to the movies, to the cleaners, to Florida, wherever, make a pact with yourself that however you go, you'll return a different way. Keep finding new ways to go to the same old places.

Go somewhere you've never been and know nothing about, and just follow your nose. For example, explore a new neighborhood, find a new trail.

Several years ago, I broke my right wrist and suddenly became left-handed—it was a revelation. Putting on my makeup, getting dressed, writing, washing my hair—everything was new. Spend one day using your non-dominant hand as the doer.

2. Space

Often when I lead groups, the room feels really crowded at the beginning. Put a couple hundred people in a workshop to dance and they tend to get territorial and start thinking there isn't enough space even when there is. Soon the belief that the room is too small fills the space until it actually does feel crowded.

By using the walking meditation and other exercises, I shift the focus to the space that is not occupied by another body or body part. Like Moses parting the waves, the crowded room suddenly opens up into empty space. Miracles can happen when each person seeks out the empty space rather than focusing on the idea that the person next to them is taking up all the room, and then grumbling and moaning about it.

One hot summer night a bunch of us went to a dance club called Tramps to hear an African band. The room was packed. The drummers came on stage one at a time till there were six of them each playing his own song. Then came the bass and the guitars, and by the time the singer joined in, the polyrhythms were irresistible. We were all so deep in our dance that the idea that we were packed in there like sardines never occured to us. We were just one big sea of gyrating hips.

Doing the walking meditation in a group is simple, just walk and seek the empty space. When you have a hundred people moving around a room, in a beat, each one changing direction as space opens up, it gets a bit chaotic. But inside *chaos* is an amazing sense of pattern and order; inside *chaos* we find our destiny. Recently a woman told me that doing this meditation changed her life. She realized that she had not been seeking the empty space in life but was always wanting what someone else had or thinking she should be where they were, instead of where she was.

A man in a workshop told me he had just come back from Katmandu where traffic was horrendous, totally *chaotic* and to his mind, rather dangerous. There were no rules or laws. After one particularly harrowing ride he asked the driver, "How do you stay alive in this traffic with no rules?" The driver giggled. "I go for the empty spaces."

To Do
(or Not To Do)

Space

Go to a club and seek the empty spaces on the dance floor, moving between the bodies like a curve of light. Make this your meditation. Or find a crowded street and move through the empty spaces, trying not to break your flow or bump into anyone. Walk in a field of high grass or move in a forest, dancing into the empty spaces as they arise.

3. Attention/Awareness/Action

> *I went into a*
> *McDonald's yesterday and*
> *said, "I'd like some fries."*
> *The girl at the counter said,*
> *"Would you like some fries*
> *with that?"*
>
> Jay Leno

Attention and awareness and action are the intelligence of the soul.

Sometimes when I'm dancing I enter an existential world where I am simply the dance; nothing more, nothing less. My body merges with the space around me until I no longer experience it as solid, but as liquid light. In this state my sense of separateness dissolves into a field of awareness. This awareness is not bound by my body; rather, my body is bound by my awareness.

Within the body, inside this field of awareness, there is a moving center, a part of me that shifts my focus—my attention. When it isn't detained elsewhere, it resides in my gut between my instincts and intuition, waiting for a signal to move. Attention is as specific as awareness is general.

It takes discipline to develop attention and awareness. For me, this discipline is part of my dance. One of the biggest challenges is to keep my awareness in my body, not in my head where it can distract me in a million ways. In the dance I practice grounding my awareness in my feet and shifting my attention to specific body parts. Ideally, attention should be a point of consciousness moving around inside the field of awareness. Awareness is the forest, attention is the trees.

As I'm dancing, my focus might gravitate toward a pain in my tooth and I can lavish as much attention on it as I want, but that won't stop it from hurting. I have to take action—call the dentist. Attention is a bridge between the receptive, feminine energy of awareness and the outgoing, masculine energy of action.

To Do
(or Not To Do)

Awareness

Wherever you are in this moment, as you continue to read and pay attention to the words on the page, become aware of your feet. If they aren't on the ground, put them there and feel the earth beneath you.

Notice how you automatically experience the motion of your breath, the tension in your shoulders, the hunger in your belly. When awareness is grounded, we become aware of what is going on in our bodies in the space between our heads and our feet.

Take a walk and keep shifting your awareness back to your feet. Remember to make this shift throughout the day; while you're standing in line for the cashier at the supermarket or at the bank, or waiting for a red light to turn green, or scrambling eggs. Find your feet.

Attention

Take inventory as you dance.

Head—What's your state of mind?
Shoulders—Do they feel tight? What are they holding?
Elbows—Follow them around the room.
Right hand—What does it want to say to you?
Left hand—Does it feel different than the right? How?
Spine—Is it loose, tight? Isolate it—lean up against the wall, lie down on the floor, move like a snake.
Chest—Sunken? Puffed out? What attitudes and feelings live here?
Hips—So many stories live here. What are yours?
Knees—Are they locked or loose? Is there any trauma? What do they have to tell?
Feet—What part of your foot do you walk on? Do you have a workout walk, ballet walk, tight-shoe-high-heel walk?

4. Breath

Breath is a promiscuous lover. The breath you just took was in someone else a moment ago, and when you let go, it'll move on and become part of someone else. Breath keeps everything moving; without it, there can be no dance.

So, dance with awareness of your breath. Pay attention to its rhythm, to the parts of you that are being breathed and the parts of you that aren't. Maybe there is no movement in a shoulder or in your pelvis; no movement means no breath. Focus on this part of you, breathe into it, and let go of whatever it is holding. Every part of us needs breath to catalyze its function.

Your breath is the most vital and important thing about you. If you don't breathe, you die. But more importantly, if you don't breathe, you can't dance.

To Do
(or Not To Do)

Awareness

The breath is the metaphor and medium of your receptivity. Close your eyes and get a sense of what's longer, your inhale or your exhale. Are you a shallow breather? A mouth breather? A no breather? Or do you breathe deeply and fully, from the bottom of your belly? Do you cut off your inhale, control how deep it goes? Your story is in the dance of your breath. Breathing is how spirit moves through matter; it's our most down-home religious movement.

Put on some uptempo music like "Snake" on my album *Bones,* and dance till you drop. Sit and watch your breath, listen to its song, tune in to it as an inner dance. It is through breathing that spirit unites with flesh. Think of them as two long-lost lovers or high-school sweethearts meeting again.

5. Music
The rhythms can be done to any kind of music—heavy metal, techno, world beat, classical, or any other style, real or imagined, as long as it turns you on. I will offer you all kinds of suggestions along the

way, but know that it's what gets your mojo working that counts. If you're clueless about music, don't worry. Be happy—I've spent the last fifteen years making music that supports this style of dancing and it's available. Often the practice is done to no music at all. Being fluid is the goal—to be absolutely fluid, to hold back nothing, to trust, and to have faith in whims, impulses, desires, and other acts of intuition.

When you choose your music, you're setting the stage for your experience—it's a conscious choice that should support what you want to do in your practice that day. Do you want it to be low-key or energetic? You may need to plug into *staccato* to get ready for a contract negotiation. So find some rock 'n' roll with a heavy 4/4 beat or whatever else takes you there, pump up the volume, and listen with your whole body to the beat.

To Do
(or Not To Do)

Music

Close the door, pull down the shades, pick out a passionate piece of music, and turn it up real loud. Now, lie down on the floor and let your body become a speaker. Listen to the music with your whole body. Listen with your head, your shoulders, your elbows, your hands, your spine, your belly, your thighs, your knees, your calves, your feet. Let the music pass through you. Feel the vibration of the music in each part of you. Which part feels the bass, the treble? What instrument tugs at your heart, your hips?

Play it again. This time, move your body—dance with this new awareness of the music.

You can use music to help you to figure out which is your dominant rhythm. Imagine your life as a silent movie and sit back and watch it. Back up a few days, watch yourself move from morning till night, doing the simple ordinary moves of your day—eating, dressing, walking, talking, waiting, wondering. To what beat do you move, what tempo? Listen to the soundtrack; what would be the most suitable music for your life story?

The Offering

The Wave is a spiritual practice, so start off with a prayer. My favorite is: "God is truly amazing. God is within me and I am within God." Then offer each of your body parts to the dance. Offer your shoulders to the dance, "Take my shoulders, use my shoulders, free my shoulders, they are yours," and then let your shoulders guide the rest of your body in a dance. Do this with elbows, hands, spine, hips, knees, feet—with every part of you. Give all of yourself to the dance: "Take me. Use me. Move me even deeper within you." Do this until your whole body awakens.

Knowing the difference between leading and following energy is crucial to your sense of balance. Some people can only lead, others can only follow. If you are stuck being a leader you need people to lead; if you're stuck being a follower you need somebody to follow. Either way is out of balance and a sure path to resentment. We need to know both to freely act in whatever mode is appropriate. In a tribe of dolphins, whoever is in front leads; when that dolphin is tired, he or she drops behind and whoever happens to be in front next leads. No attachment. No elections. No politics. We aren't like dolphins but we could be, at least in the context of our own psyches. In this discipline, we practice being both leader and follower, letting one part of our body lead while the rest follows. That way we can "know the masculine and keep to the feminine," as the *Tao Te Ching* advises.

In trance dancing, any part of your body may lead you into ecstasy—your hand, your hips. When you are lost in the dance, the beat will call to different parts of you, and if you have trained yourself to listen and follow your body parts, you will hear and you will follow and you will be danced.

Dance till you sweat.
Then, dance some more.
Do it alone.
Do it with others.
Do it often.
Do it with attitude.
Do it with an attitude of prayer.

Do you have the discipline to be a free spirit?

Chapter Three

THE ARCHETYPES

Nothing worse could
happen to one than to be
completely understood.
C. G. Jung

T he rhythms, when I first identified and named them, turned
out to be much more than a
way to work out my body. They became a way to work out my soul—
to sensitize my intuition, stretch my imagination, and tap new levels of
inspiration that I had never dreamed existed. Each rhythm was a state
of being; an outrageous world of deep inner teachings on the nature of
life and love, birth and death, art and God. Each rhythm awakened energies that helped me to separate myself from my conditioning, dis-

cover my original passions and desires, and connect me to my humanity. The rhythms gave me a way to map the movements of my own psyche as well as the ever-changing state of the universe. In their context, I was able to grasp my feminine roots, spread my masculine wings, and traverse the world with winged feet.

Dancing each of the five rhythms transported me into a different state of being and revealed a different aspect of my true self. I was excited by my discovery, but stumped as to how to communicate it to others so that they, too, could explore these hidden realms of the soul. I needed a language, a vocabulary of images, that would be clear and accessible without being restrictive or reductive. I began to play around with some of the archetypes most evocative and familiar to me: *mother, mistress, madonna, father, son,* and *holy spirit.* The first three reflected the different energy fields mapped by the feminine rhythm of *flowing,* while the latter three correlated with the energies I felt when dancing the masculine rhythm of *staccato.*

I had to begin in zero and forget everything I knew about these words. It's the misuse and abuse of them that has caused us two thousand years of pain, separating spirit from flesh, body from soul, and sexuality from sacredness. So first I stripped the archetypes of all religious content to look at them in their purity, to feel their original spirit, to find the dance behind the dogma. When I conceived of *son,* I wasn't thinking about Jesus or my beautiful son Jonny, but the wild part of my soul, the part of me that could hang out in a desert for forty days and forty nights, rage against the machine, or sacrifice anything for inner freedom.

As I began to use these archetypes in my teaching, I ran into a problem: people took them too literally, locking in on a single stereotypic meaning for each, reducing them to mere characters. I had to explain that the archetypes were just metaphors and should not be interpreted too rigidly. The point of choosing Judeo-Christian archetypes is not to play into their firmly established cultural constructs, but to take advantage of how deeply ingrained they are in us. These words evoke instant, viceral feelings that bypass the brain and hit us right in the gut. If

I were from an Indian or Chinese or African background, I'd have chosen archetypes common to those cultures.

The divine is by definition a mystery beyond our powers of com-
prehension. Paradoxically, it is within our grasp if we approach it with
innocence. As Einstein queried, "Why is it that I get my best ideas in
the morning while I'm shaving?" Shaving is like meditation with a
sharp object. When the mind is empty and receptive, big ideas flow
through every cell of our body. When we're thinking too hard, we
tense up and nothing can flow through us; our energy gets stuck in our
heads. Sometimes you have to take a leap of faith and trust that if you
turn off your head, your feet will take you where you need to go.

In a way, the archetypes chose me, I didn't choose them. I wasn't
shaving, I was dancing, and they fell into my consciousness. I couldn't
figure them out intellectually, but I knew on an instinctive level that
they were tracks to the divine mystery. I followed these tracks in my
dance, some led me to my masculine soul, some to my feminine soul.
And in the alchemical wedding of all of them, I discovered that my
soul was truly androgynous.

People have the hardest time understanding the differences among
the feminine archetypes. I think it's because it seems as if there are
only two. The *mother* is the *madonna*, right? Actually, wrong. If you
read between the lines, you'll notice that there are, in fact, three distinct Marys: Mary, *mother* of Jesus; Mary Magdalene, *mistress* of Jesus—
I don't mean to imply that he put her up in the Bethlehem Hilton;
rather that, as *mistress*, she represents the wilderness of the heart; and
Mary, sister of Lazarus and Martha, who sat at His feet, absorbing His
stories and wisdom. This third Mary embodies the contemplative energies of *madonna*. These three Marys represent his body, his heart,
and his mind, as they do ours.

The holy trinity of the feminine soul has been reduced to a dichotomy: virgin or whore. In *A History of God*, Karen Armstrong
suggests that the point of trinities is that they're beyond the grasp of
the human mind and inherently mysterious. On the other hand, dichotomies are the patterns of the everyday: good and evil, black and

white, male and female. By reducing the feminine trinity to a dichotomy, it is robbed of its divine power. This has had a tragic effect on both men and women, taking the sacredness out of our sexuality and leaving women corseted into extreme and clichéd patterns of behavior and men with nothing but a hole where their feminine consciousness should be.

So when I discuss the *mother* archetype, for example, I'm not talking about June Cleaver, Roseanne, or Hillary Rodham Clinton. I'm talking about you, and your challenge is to discover the original way this archetype manifests in your soul. *Mother* is a gateway to an energy field which contains a multitude of characters embodying many different qualities. While the teen *mother* has to remember to take her pill, the crone *mother* has to remember to take her estrogen. Mother Hubbard, Mother England, Mother Superior, and Mommie Dearest all inhabit this archetypal realm. Gender isn't an issue, either: little girls tap into their *mother* energies when they play with their dolls, just as little boys do when they take care of their puppies and big boys do when they comfort their lovers.

Chaos is the rhythm in which we integrate our masculine and feminine energies, so it made sense that the archetypes of *chaos* should reflect the creative energy of that union. *Artist* is the archetype I chose to represent the marriage of *mother* and *father*. *Lover* represents the mutual seduction of *mistress* and *son*. And *seeker* reflects the communion of *madonna* and *holy spirit*.

The archetype for the *lyrical* rhythm is the *shapeshifter*, an embodiment of the universal dynamic of change. In this domain we can transform ourselves, drawing on different archetypal energies whenever we need them. These needs arise all the time in our day-to-day lives. When I'm teaching, for example, I draw heavily on *mother*, who tracks the physical energy of the room, making sure everyone is comfortable. Is it too hot? Should we open some windows? People seem tired today, I think I'll juice them up with some hard-core rock n' roll. At the same time, the *mistress* part of me tracks the room's emotional energy. *Mistress* is also the energy I use to seduce people into the dance and, once they're dancing, ever deeper into their bodies. *Madonna* is responsible for maintaining a sense of the sacredness of the whole process. She listens for feedback and encourages people to keep their minds empty, free of distracting dogma.

My masculine energies are also in play. *Father* sets the boundaries and rules: no gum, no alcohol, no talking. *Son* counters this by pushing people to take risks and dance on the edge, keeping things from getting too soft and safe. Meanwhile, my *holy spirit* works to keep us moving toward the higher self, the deep and divine space we're seeking together. As *shapeshifter*, I can switch in and out of these energies in an instant, balancing an awareness of the whole with attention to specific details so that I can take the right actions.

Sometimes energy fields feel a little like quicksand—we get stuck in a particular archetype and experience its shadow side and the negative emotions that go with it. We've all had these moments—when mothering turns into smothering, when flirtation becomes obsession, when playfulness escalates into dangerous behavior. A teacher who's stuck in *mother* will infantalize her students, while one stuck in *mistress* will view them all as potential conquests. A young friend of mine complained that her mother was driving her crazy—the woman is a therapist and insists on analyzing everything her daughter says or does. She's stuck in *madonna*. *Father* can get overbearing, while *son* can get out of control. Even too much *holy spirit* can be a bad thing—think of the person with a missionary complex who treats everyone they meet as a potential convert.

We all have the potential to be a full-bodied Bordeaux, but sadly most of us are satisfied being Welch's grape juice.

Sometimes we put all our eggs in one archetype and live one-dimensionally. I know a man with a formidable *mistress*. I call him Tantra-Man. Perhaps you've met him—he gets around. Tantra-Man knows who he is and is perfectly clear in his non-attachment. Why do we always believe we're the exception?

Or, how about the sex kitten who slinks into the room purring "hello," rubs up against you and makes you aware of that insatiable itch. She's in her body and is not ashamed to share it; feels her emotions and is not afraid to show them. She's considered a predator when in fact she's just preening. Your body is her temple.

Other people are underdeveloped in a particular archetypal energy. You can cultivate that side with a little help from your friends. The seed is there; God planted it. We all contain the entire spectrum, but often one or more energies have been depressed, repressed, suppressed—all the pressed words—to the point where we believe they aren't inherent in each of us.

My husband, Robert, had weak *mother* energy so I bought him a cat to ignite it. A guy I know was dating a woman whose wild *son* was M.I.A., so he insisted she learn how to Rollerblade and ski before he'd pop the question. My girlfriend, "Dolly Doormat," has no sense of *father*, so after her last lover left his imprint on her chest, we sent her to a Tae Kwon Do class.

We tend to attract people who fill our holes. I know a young stockbroker, in whom everything is linear, reduced to money. He works out at the gym, parties every night with the guys, and golfs on the weekends, but there's no sense of the sacred in anything he is or does. He doesn't believe there is anything bigger than him. And so his subconscious balanced him out by leading him to marry a practicing Orthodox Jew.

Then there's the guy who's driven by his wild *son*. Everything is out of control: his emotions run wild; he lives on the edge, bungee-jumping, driving with a beer between his legs, always pushing the limits. He's so wonderfully irresponsible you can't pin him down to anything—including his own opinions. So, he falls in love with an earth-mother type, Birkenstocks and all, who immediately gets pregnant. The baby brings out his nurturing *mother* which then grounds his wildness a bit.

I know a woman with a teaching credential who can't make a living in this world because she doesn't live in it, she only dreams about it. Of course, reality never measures up to her fantasies, which drives her further into her own darkness and despair. She has a completely atrophied *father*, no wild *son*, a weak *mother* and an absentee *mistress*. The *madonna* and *holy spirit* star in her movie. She seeks balance by always attaching herself to lovers who have strong *father* energy, capable and competent in the world, with a hint of wild *son*.

The archetype responsible for getting us unstuck, for partnering us in our shadow dance and leading us into the light, is the *alchemist*. In the realm of *stillness*, the *alchemist* turns lead into gold, healing our psychic wounds and repairing the damage done to our souls by the destructive forces of ego.

When ego is directing the show, we're mere character actors. When the soul is empowered, we have an infinite repertoire of possible roles. We are huge; the only thing that limits us is our own narrow minds— our fixed ideas of who we are and our fears of innovation and experimentation. In spite of what Shakespeare says, none of us is merely "a poor player who struts and frets his hour upon the stage and then is heard no more." We are the whole theater company—actors, director, producer, costume designer, lighting engineer, ticket agent—and we can choose what we want to perform on any given night: comedy or tragedy, drama or romance. If you're true to yourself and practice all the parts, every performance can be the performance of a lifetime.

When you are in your soul, when you are coming from that place of being connected with your essence, you are in touch with all aspects of yourself. And the alchemy of these attributes that you carry within you—unique and constantly shifting—will forever be a mystery. But it is a mystery worth investigating for the rest of your life. Out of the mix, which each of us embodies, and within which each of us is embodied, come the mysterious dynamics of *you*, your essence.

To sum up, in the rhythm of *flowing* we receive the feminine teachings, in *staccato* we explore the masculine, in *chaos* we integrate the two. *Lyrical* is the rhythm of self-realization, in which we experience our most expansive and liberated self. In *stillness*, we contemplate the mystery that infuses every aspect of the universe—including the deepest recesses of our own souls.

Like the I Ching, the soul is fluid and everchanging. And the archetypal realms within the soul are not defined by rigid characters, conventions or boundaries. Dichotomies are static, but as soon as you add

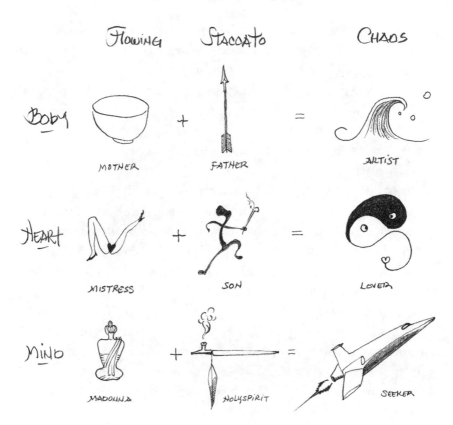

a third element, the whole system begins to move. The feminine energies are rooted in awareness; the masculine energies are about action. We need a catalyst to establish a dynamic equilibrium between them and in this case that catalyst is attention.

After describing each archetype, I've provided a three-part "TO DO (or NOT TO DO)." The first is a meditation to create awareness and get you thinking. The second is an action to deepen your practice. The third will help you shift your attention beyond the boundaries of yourself to the outside world by doing service or throwing a party celebrating the aspect of the soul that is the focus of that section. In the following chapters as you work your way through the five rhythms, keep in mind that they aren't only a way to view your life as energy in motion, but a spiritual practice for body and soul.

The soul is beyond description; it can't be pinned down like a but-

Lyrical

SOUL

SHAPESHIFTER

MOTHER

MISTRESS

MADONNA

FATHER

SON

HOLYSPIRIT

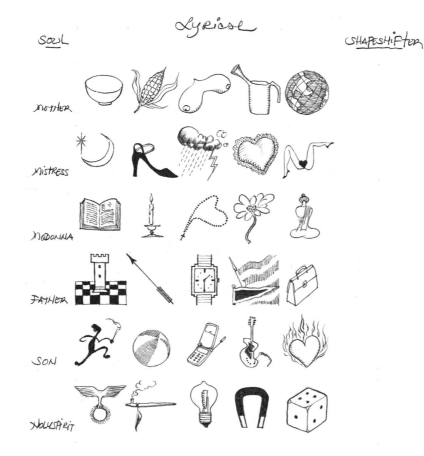

STILLNESS

SPIRIT

ALCHEMIST

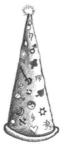

terfly in a collector' s case. But I thought it would be fun and helpful to spark your imagination with a visual map of the territory we are covering. Since no one has ever accused me of having good hand/eye coordination, I called my friend Hans, master draftsman, and gave him the assignment.

Notice that when you get to the *lyrcial* map the soul has moved into *shapeshifter* mode and the possibilities are infinite. Don't let these icons intimidate you. You don't have to "understand" them; they're meant to work below the mind as, in fact, the archetypes do. Feel free to let your mind wander and come up with your own personal set of images.

The Search for the Feminine in My Bones

I collected them all, found every bone
except I couldn't find my hand, my hand
my mother had it
her calloused hard hitting hands have held me
gripping my spirit
she seized my hand at six
stripped it of innocence and grace
she severed my hand at seven
I found it again in a dry riverbed pointing North
this hand that has the most number of bones
fragments of bones, joints and articulation
I can't open it
I have my hand now
I can pray
I can pray again
I turn to the Goddess, pray for forgiveness
She says "there is no forgiveness because there are no sins"
She places God on the tips of my fingers
on the tips of my toes
and tells me that everyone has to learn how to pray
in their own way
in their own way with everything, everywhere
I collected them all, found every splintered bone
every piece of myself
now I dance flinging my bones to the floor
like the I Ching
like the I Ching each time I hit the floor
I'm different

Jewel Mathieson

Chapter Four

FLOWING

kite moving through sky
Great Wall of China
weeping willow bending in the
  wind
wheat waving in wind
telemark skiing
tai chi
wolf howl
Argentinian tango
Whoopi Goldberg
putting on hand cream
time lapse photography
Van Gogh, *Starry Night*
Grace Kelly
TWA's terminal at JFK
glass elevators traveling
  upwards
fly fishing
Isadora Duncan
The Guggenheim Museum
the smooth panning of a 75mm
  movie camera
shadow of clouds rolling across
  the landscape
single autumn leaf falling from
  maple tree

Hanna Schygulla
toilet paper being flushed
surfing
sailing
dolphins
hula
Michelangelo, *The Creation of
  Adam*
weaving
silk velvet
ice skating
Botticelli's *Venus*
the swelling skirt of a dancing
  dervish
eagle in flight
calligraphy
French
desert dunes
Gaudi's architecture
the scroll stock index at the
  bottom of your TV screen (turn
  your channel to Headline News)
the twisted columns and
  sweeping stairways at St.
  Peter's

O
n Sundays it seems the whole
world slows down, even New
York City, this crazy place I call
home. After twenty years of togetherness, Robert and I have our Sunday ritual down. He jumps up, showers, and goes on the bread-and-
paper hunt while I roll out of bed, boil the water and heat the milk for

coffee, choose the mood music, trim the flowers and change their water. Just as I finish, he returns with a bag filled with goodies from the neighborhood gourmet shop. I make tea while he does his coffee thing, and then we each take "our" sections of the paper and lose ourselves in a world of words.

Today we decided that breakfast was just an appetizer for brunch, so we headed down to Soho to a little restaurant on West Broadway. The hostess led us deep into the dark, close, cavelike room. Wine bottles lined the burgundy brick walls, ceiling fans slowly whirled like lost birds above us. Everything and everyone seemed to be moving to a laid-back Euro-disco beat.

I emerged into the daylight in a spaghetti arrabiata–induced spell, feeling all warm and spicy inside. All the sharp edges seemed to be blurred and my eye picked up only softness and curves: a row of banners floating above the boutiques like French can-can dancers, the European woman walking in front of me in buttery leather pants, the fluffy white poodle peeking out of her husband's backpack, the ancient man hunched over his synthesizer with an upturned bowler hat in front of him for donations.

A colorful painting in a window grabbed my attention, so I breezed into the gallery for a closer look. It was an oil painting of a luscious tangerine-colored nude with hot-pink nipples and livid purple hair. She was reclining with her knees up and legs crossed, the lush curves of her body a celebration of the feminine spirit. Everything about her was sensuous, hot, earthy, and inviting. I noted that all of this artist's female nudes were bold and curvaceous, reveling in the juicy joy of being in their bodies.

We meandered in the direction of Canal Street on our way to the flea market. Once again I was seduced off course, however; this time by a bright yellow banner depicting a blue dog with yellow eyes and a white nose. It was staring down at me from a gallery across the street which was holding an exhibit of "Blue Dog" paintings. The story behind the paintings was that the artist had a dog named Tiffany, a cross between a spaniel and terrier. When she died, he couldn't stop dreaming about her, and so he began to paint her. As I left I noticed a quote written on the window. "To find her you must lose her. The Blue Dog knows the way."

We rounded the corner and wafted into an exhibit of photos by Peter Beard. Another nude woman, this one feeding a giraffe something from a large oval leaf, maybe water. They resembled one another, the woman and the giraffe, the bend of their long, slender necks. All of the images focused on the intersection—either violent or beautiful—between human and animal kingdoms. Alternately majestic and humble, the pictures enthralled me. We lingered so long in the gallery that when we finally emerged, we'd missed the flea market entirely. It was time to start thinking about dinner.

We decided to go to the River Cafe in Brooklyn. Seated by the window, we gazed out at a symphony of *flowing* images. Barges, tugs, and sailboats cruised the East River. Cars streamed north and south on the FDR Drive. Planes circled La Guardia, etching arcs of light in the indigo sky. And over everything loomed the magnificent curved suspension of the great Brooklyn Bridge, like the Great Mother embracing her two shores.

Flowing is the state of being fluid, of hanging loose and being flexible. The rhythm of *flowing* connects us to the flow of our individual energy, our base current. When we dance long and hard enough to cast off the world's spell, our inner rhythm takes over and we begin to sense who we truly are and how great our potential is. To my mind, Michael Jordan playing basketball is the essence of *flowing*. His internal rhythm connects with the energies of the ball, his team, his opponents, and the court, until they all merge into one organic entity and it becomes as natural for the ball to swoosh through the net as it is for breath to flow in and out of our bodies.

When we're in our flow, all we have to do is walk across a room to be mesmerizing. We feel confident in ourselves because we're connected to the earth and in harmony with her rhythms, cycles, and moods. In *flowing,* there are no separations or distinctions between things, there's only continuous change. We tend to resist surrendering to this rhythm because we prefer life to be predictable and safe, even if it means being bored. *Flowing* is dangerous—who knows where it will take you or what you will find when you get there? That's why I love it.

Flowing is the rhythm of the earth. Some people are in tune with her, some are not, but all of us are subject to her ups and downs. She seems to be in a rather volatile mood these days—I find myself glued to the Weather Channel, tracking her turbulent patterns. Perhaps she's avenging the neglect, misuse, and abuse that we have inflicted upon her. These natural disasters remind us how vulnerable we are to the flow of her energy, how connected we are to her cycles, how dependent we are on her gifts.

In a room full of diverse, sweaty dancers practicing the *flowing* rhythm, I recognize the motions of the earth as the bodies orbit each other and spin on their own axes. The energy builds and the room transforms into a womb, rocking in rhythmic contractions; a sea of bodies tossing up limbs in flashes of flesh and snatches of color. It doesn't start out this way, of course. Sometimes I find myself faced with a wall of inertia. Looking out over a heap of bodies dragged down by all their baggage, I feel like a lone porter at JFK during rush hour. I know we're eventually going to take off—my faith is grounded in experience—but sometimes we get fogged in for a while by judgments and longings, resentments and comparisons, vanity and depression. This negative energy actually weighs something, so I usually start by having everybody dance their heaviness, knowing that on the other side of it is light.

My eyes scan the dancing bodies but keep returning to a young man. He's been gliding along the surface doing his standard repetoire of *flowing* moves, when suddenly something shifts inside of him. He transcends his boredom and enters the body of a panther on Rollerblades. Moves spin out from his center in endless waves, some breathtaking to watch. He disappears in the dance until all that's left of him is a mop of bleached-white hair in a torn black t-shirt and jeans. He tracks dreams, despair, and dirty dances back to their source in gutsy, instinct-driven, raunchy rolls. He dissolves in a swirl of arms, in the sweep of a leg, in the curve of his neck. His eyes turn inward, his feet listening to the songs of the Great Mother emanating from the sprung-wood floor beneath him. He surrenders his bones to the waves and dances in the ocean of his being.

The teachings of *flowing* unfold organically in the dancing body. In this rhythm we sense our connection to the birth cycle and return to a prelogical, intuitive state, as if we were infants again, eagerly and unself-consciously absorbing the world around us. In that stage of life, Nature is hip enough to provide us with time to get used to being in bodies, to get grounded on this earth, in our instincts, in the flow of our energy. She provides us with time to bond with the mother—the one inside, the one outside, and the Great Mother who nurtures us all.

My friends Kathy and Lori have wanted a baby for the last ten years. Finally, they've been blessed with Daniel. Shortly after they brought him home from the hospital, in response to my eager curiosity about the baby, Kathy faxed me a page from her journal.

"Like the weather map on the 11 o'clock news, I watch the myriad of expressions speed across my son's face. There's more information in his 30-second soundbites than the best copyeditor can conjure. He goes from frowning, laughing, crying, and smiling to simply staring at the angels clearly within his view; flowing through states of being free of evaluation, justification, or the need to please. He feels his gas and bears down, purple-faced, to shit. He grunts and whines, and when the shit passes, he's asleep on the exhale.

"In these eight short weeks I have learned more about the power of just being from my 12-pounder (yes, that's smaller than a Thanksgiving turkey) than in 20 years of practicing my flow. But it is not lost on me that all this practice has readied me for the shock of having to surrender my life to his flow."

We're all born immersed in the universal flow, but as we grow into kids we get socialized, intellectualized, homogenized, and often cut off from the source. Growing up isn't what it was cracked up to be. Sadly, it usually requires us to disconnect from our primal natures, our sensual selves. Different things cut us off—panic, overexertion, self-consciousness, laziness, worry, and stress are all *flow* freezers.

Alienated from our own instincts, we lose both our ability to be aware and our ability to pay attention. In my teaching I see people every day who have no idea that they're tired, hungry, frustrated, lonely, bored, or sad. They're completely out of touch with themselves, nor do they pay attention to anyone else. This state of unconsciousness is like living in a ghost town from some fifth-rate Czechoslovakian cowboy flick—all facades and tumbleweed, only nobody's riding through town.

Because mind is matter, this somnambulent state is reflected in our bodies. When I think I'm worthless, my chest sinks and my head hangs forward. The body never lies.

In *flowing,* we learn how to inhale, how to take things in: compliments, put-downs, gifts, intuitive hunches, moods, music, space— whoever or whatever else is going on around us. We like to delude ourselves that we're encased in an impermeable membrane floating through life in our own little space capsule. We think we're so self-sufficient, but actually we're all just passing thoughts in one huge universal mind.

Flowing is more than a rhythm; it's a specific energy field in which the feminine aspect of the soul is revealed in all its awesome beauty, fierce power, and animal magnetism. Deep within each one of us is a *mother* longing to nurture, a *mistress* impatient to flirt, and a *madonna* serene in her wisdom. And they all bop out when the beat kicks in.

TO DO (or NOT TO DO)—*Flowing*

Feel your feet rooted into the ground. On the inhale, let your breath lift your arms. As you exhale, lower them. Continue rising on the inhale and sinking on the exhale. Focus on your belly button. Expand from your belly on the inhale and contract into your belly on the exhale. Open your whole body like a poppy, then close it down as if it were night. Do these movements in sync with your breath. One movement merges and melts into the next. Let your feet move; follow your feet around the room (don't forget to keep your eyes open), changing the tempo but never interrupting your flow. Dance as if you were moving through honey.

Imagine you are all circles and curves, arms round, spine undulating, hands soft, hips rolling gently, knees loose. Allow your body to weave an endless stream of circles—powerful, relaxed, earthy. Surrender to your feet, each part of you partnering with your feet—elbows and feet, shoulders and feet, hands and feet—having dialogues in space.

Let whatever you are feeling unravel. Don't force it—you don't need to make any effort, just let them flow. Sense the space around you and move with it as if it were your lover.

Breathe the whole world into yourself. Rising and sinking. Letting go. Following the flow of your energy.

Suggested music:

SONG	ALBUM	COMMENT
"Persephone's Song"	Luna	slow
"Prairie Ruins"	Ritual	medium
"Jamu"	Zone Unknown	fast

Mother

As you are, so is the world.

Ramana Maharshi

I'm a downtown kind of gal, but I was in such agony the other day that I made a pilgrimage to the Upper West Side to get a Lomi Ka'Ala Hoku massage. I arrived at Eōlani's building in one piece—no mean feat, as most of New York's cabdrivers have learner's permits issued in Bangladesh. As the tiny elevator creaked up the nine floors, I talked myself down from an anxiety attack; having survived an elevator mishap a few years ago I am now certifiably claustrophobic in shaky ones. As soon as it stopped, I leaped out and rang her bell.

Eōlani opened the door and I passed into another world. Although still on the island of Manhattan, everything in her apartment was reminiscent of Hawaii, including the temperature. A multicolored fish mobile gently swayed over the sink, a statue of Memaya, the Yoruba goddess of the ocean, guarded the refrigerator, and a minature fountain bubbled behind the curtain of her massage room. Eōlani looked like a bird of paradise in her sarong. As I was getting undressed, a cheeky little gray-and-white cockatiel with orange cheeks and a yellow crown landed on my head.

I gratefully climbed on the table and surrendered to the sound of recorded waves as Eōlani stood beside me and said a prayer for my healing. "Beloved Creator, Blessed Mother, we call upon you and ask that your presence be felt here now. Bless and guide this session with Gabrielle. May Love, Light, and Healing pour through us and may the ripples of this session flow out to all beings and to our Beloved Mother Earth." Amen.

In Lomi Lomi massage the hands never leave the body, the circle is unbroken, and the rhythm is continuous. The waves faded out to tribal drums overlaid with Hawaiian chants as Eōlani's forearms kneaded and rolled across the landscape of my body. She lifted and cradled me, rocking me in the arms of the *mother,* sweeping me into her grace. I became wide open and receptive. In the spirit of Aloha, unconditional love, I felt like a newborn babe, soft and silky.

When the massage was over, I descended the nine floors oblivious to the shimmying elevator and floated out to the sidewalk. It was a rainy spring day. The taxi drove through the park, past runners, lovers, dog walkers, and the topiary gorilla at Tavern on the Green, and out on to Seventh Avenue. I felt as if I were in a musical with all the colored umbrellas bobbing along the streets. My taxi was a magic carpet; traffic seemed to disappear as soon as we approached. As we cruised by the Carnegie Deli, I recalled all the times I used to go there for cheese

blintzes whenever I felt like I needed the comfort of a mother. We blew
through Times Square, where I waved to Kate Moss and the sexy Perry
Ellis couple on the billboards. According to the Viacom Spectra color
screen the time was 4:10 and the temperature was 56. It's always cool to
know how hot it is. The Virgin Records Megastore was the last thing to
catch my eye before we entered a wasteland of nondescript gray buildings. We sped past showrooms and trucks unloading racks of dresses,
culminating in Macy's, purportedly The World's Largest Store. At Her-
ald Square we hit a traffic jam that only the delivery boys on bikes
could penetrate. I reminded myself that the end of one *flow* is the beginning of another.

A young girl hobbled past the taxi on crutches. It immediately reminded me of my son Jonathan and the devastating snowboard accident that blew out his right knee. The surgeon told us that he had
repaired thousands of knees and this was the worst he had ever seen.

"It caused a dramatic awakening of my inner *mother*," Jonny later
told me. "Suddenly I was thrust into a whole new state of consciousness. I couldn't move without being aware of every step, every shift of
my weight. I had to learn to love myself when I wasn't perfect and
keep my mind focused on my healing instead of on all that I was missing. Cooking lunch took up a major part of my day. I was so sad—I
couldn't even watch a sentimental commercial without crying. I could
be in rehab riding my bike or trying to maneuver my way up the stairs
and I'd just start crying. My emotions had all sorts of room to move
and my ego had no control over them.

"I spent my days with Kaya, Todd's golden Labrador retriever. I was
reduced to the life of a dog. I'd go out and smoke a cigarette, throw a
frisbee, he'd catch it. We'd sniff around the house for a while, lie on the
couch and have some doggie dreams, and then Todd would come
home and feed us. I was so happy to have a friend on the same level as
I was.

"I was used to living a wild, energetic, active life; now everything
was slow motion. It took me an hour to take a shower. My life was suddenly very Zen."

The light had changed a dozen times by now and we hadn't moved an inch, so I got out and walked the last mile home in long, lopey strides. I reflected on how this accident had both transformed my son into a man and initiated that man into the deeper mysteries of the *mother*.

During a *God, Sex, and the Body* workshop George confided that although he understood the concept of the inner *mother* intellectually, he hadn't experienced her until his divorce. "I didn't like my own mother, so I had no positive role model for how to mother myself. Besides, for more than twenty years my wife took care of all that. Then, all of a sudden, I was on my own. Even the most mundane chores, like cooking and doing the laundry, were powerful medicine for me. Now it feels good to have a drawer full of clothes I put there myself—they didn't just mystically appear."

Even though I'm a woman, I sometimes lose touch with my internal *mother*, as well. Recently I was sitting on my couch staring into space, preoccupied and paralyzed by the stack of unopened mail sitting on the ottoman. I felt as if there were a person trapped inside each envelope judging me for not answering them, but I couldn't move. The sound of the fax machine startled me out of my misery. It was from Lorca, a gorgeous young actress friend of mine. "I thought you might need some inspiration," she had scribbled across page one. How could she possibly have known my stuck state of being? It was a letter her mom had written to her:

Lorca baby,
You always strive forward, in spite of setbacks or rewards. The *I Ching* says, "Perseverance furthers." Perseverance implies MOTION, not a sedentary state of self-centerness. To persevere means to make a move, to keep going. Yes, it's okay to stop for contemplation and meditation and prayer and a regrouping of your inner items, but that stopping becomes an impetus for INSPIRATION, so that the creative process can be renewed again and again!
    I'm just saying we love you, always and forever, unceasing. That's all.
                                                                              Mom

How could this woman sitting in a black rocker in the middle of Texas know precisely what I needed to hear? But then I remembered she hadn't written it to me. I picked up the phone and dialed Lorca's number and asked, "What's going on? Why did your mother write you this letter?"

She told me she had been struggling with an overbearing, super-critical director and had suffered a lapse of self-confidence so she called her mom. "That's wild," I said, "because you faxed it to me at exactly the moment when I needed a hit of that mom energy. I had lost faith in my ability to answer my own mail."

A mother in Fort Worth, Texas, writes a letter to her kid in North Carolina and it ends up on my lap in Manhattan on an almost spring day. The circle keeps turning. The grace of the universal *mother* keeps flowing, reminding us to return to that state of childlike innocence whenever the world becomes so overwhelming that we lose our connection to our true selves.

Greg called and told me his friend Carol was falling apart and felt like she was losing her soul, so he decided to make her dinner. He put on a dress, an apron, and some lipstick, and whipped up a lavish meal. When she arrived, he opened the door and said, "You need a mother."

After dinner they went to a funky dance club and danced to South African music all night long. It's the kind of music that hips find irresistible; it rocks them into its *flowing* vibe, into the belly of the beat, where they meet the divine *mother*. It takes you right down to that place inside you where nothing is fixed and everything moves in waves, down to the zone of survival tactics and necessary instincts you need to draw on if you want to surrender to your soul. Surrender is the password that unlocks doors into other dimensions and allows you to get past yourself and keep going.

I used to go to a belly-dance studio in midtown Manhattan, one flight up and worlds removed from the pressures of the city. It was the only place I knew where the more flesh you had the better.

In this room, all different kinds of women met to shed their skins and to unite in a deep, ancient, terrifyingly familiar desire—a strange, haunting call back to their primordial selves. Sinuous music seduced us with its hypnotic charm into worlds we hungered to know, worlds within us still untouched by the great male hunters, virgin worlds.

I stood in the doorway transfixed by the vision of a lone student, a woman in her seventies, being coaxed into her pelvis for the first time. At first she was a rock of resistance; thousands of beliefs and attitudes stiffened her body. I knew them. I felt them. Slowly she made the descent into her hips, into the beat. Another fallen woman, I thought, with a serene smile on her face.

The aspect of the soul that is *mother* lives in your hips and grounds you in an earthy, instinctive way. Not to be grounded is to be like an uprooted tree. On the subway, on the street, in airports, I look for bodies with an assured sense of self, a rootedness, a flow, an acceptance, maybe even a dash of self-love. More often than not, I see something else: the body as motherless child.

For many of us, it's a struggle to integrate the basics. We're too busy; we have more important things to do, places to be, people to see, mountains to climb. We get so caught up in our heads we trip over our own feet. I had an investment banker in my last workshop who was famous for his ability to manage the flow of huge sums of money, but he couldn't manage the flow of his own energy across the room. Overweight and out of breath, he stumbled and gasped his way through the rhythms. By the end of the five days he was no longer wheezing and there was the beginning of a spring in his step.

There is a part of us that knows what we need and when we need it. The voice of *mother*, reminding us to eat our veggies, get our teeth cleaned, and never say, "I told you so."

> *What a strange*
> *machine man is! You fill*
> *him with bread, wine, fish,*
> *and radishes, and out come*
> *sighs, laughter, and dreams.*
> Nikos Kazantzakis

Mother tends the fire in the belly. No mama, no *chi*. A student of mine was abusing alcohol during a stressful period of her life. She went to a Chinese doctor and he told her that if she kept up her drinking her *chi* would be gone in a year. When she looked at him blankly, he said, "No *chi*, no life."

Our roots are matriarchal. We come out of our mother's body and are nurtured by Mother Earth. The blood of the *mother* runs in our veins; her spirit is in all things. She can hold us in bondage or liberate us. It is up to us.

Mother is the cornerstone for all the other archetypes. Without her presence, they have no support. She is bottom-line. Her presence provides the solid ground upon which we can build the dance itself. Like the mother of our physical birth, she is the assembly point where all the mysterious forces of our being converge and manifest.

TO DO (or NOT TO DO)—*Mother*

Awareness

Make a cup of tea and sit someplace comfortable to contemplate your own universe. Begin with your body. Focus your attention on your blood. It's the most fluid thing about you; you can't hold on or control it like your breath. It's been circulating for centuries in your bloodlines, through your ancestors. It's the key to your story—past, present, and future. What is that story?

Action

Do the rhythm of *flowing* in slow motion, feeling the weight of your head, your shoulders, your arms, your hands, your chest, your hips, your legs. Surrender this weight to your feet and let them glide across the floor as they hold your weight. After a while, lie down on the floor and give your weight to the floor. Move with the floor as if it were a lover. Roll onto one side and let all your liquids flow into that side. Roll onto another part of your body and feel the liquid shift, as if there were undulating waves within you. Keep slowly rolling and releasing, allowing your fluidity to inform your dance. Try this with a lover, rolling around their curves, swimming in the same pool of energy.

Mother Party

Give a party to nurture the senses. Invite your friends to dress in their most *flowing* attire and bring their favorite comfort foods and sweets—macaroni and cheese, chicken soup, blintzes, bread pudding, pies of all kinds.

As your guests enter, anoint them with scented oils. Play *flowing* sensual music. Set up a massage corner for foot and hand massage. Make sure you have incense, flowers, candles, refreshing liquids—everything you need to create a nurturing environment.

Mistress

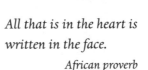

*All that is in the heart is
written in the face.*
African proverb

When something happens that shakes our very foundations, the world as we know it stops. For my son, the trauma of his knee accident put him solidly in feminine territory, where he became totally responsive to his own inner life with very few distractions. While the spirit of *mother* arose in him, so did the spirit of *mistress,* and he became as receptive to the flow of his emotional energy through the movements of his heart as he had been to the flow of his physical energy through the movements of his body. Living in slow motion, he got in touch with his sorrow—not only that linked to his present situation, but that which he had been carrying around for a long time. We don't have to understand our feelings or pin them down to specific incidents to process them. It's more important simply to let them go.

Jonny's snowboarding accident was a major event for me, as well. First there was the phone call: "He crashed into a tree on his board." I felt as if God had punched me in the stomach. I sat on my bed immobile, stunned and barely breathing. My eyes latched on to the golden Buddha hanging on the wall. I felt utterly helpless. I was reduced to shivering nerves, numb hands, and a spooked stomach. The part of me staring at the Buddha declared, "You're in terror, babe. Get a grip." I made all the necessary calls and arrangements and then, rather than give in to my helplessness, went directly to my CD collection and put on Mickey Hart's *At the Edge* with the intention of moving all this petrified energy.

Fear froze my face, my feet, my hands, my body. I had that metallic taste in my mouth that I associate with police cars in my rearview mirror. Movement was not forthcoming, but I couldn't permit myself to remain inert, so I began to sculpt myself into the pulsing, trembling shapes of my fear. As I fiercely exaggerated them, the shapes became more dynamic. I imagined Rodin turning me inside out. Slowly the shapes began dissolving into each other and becoming a heavy flowing dance. Through the simple eloquence of gesture, I finally achieved a state of calm.

Of course, there was even more stormy weather ahead. Two days later I was anxiously pacing the waiting room of the hospital as Jonny underwent his surgery. He didn't come up as expected at 5:00 P.M. By 7:30, I was back where I started, but this time there was no Buddha to offer me solace. I prowled the halls, a huge mother cat, scared to death that if I sat still the world would stop. I couldn't get anybody to answer my questions beyond the generic, "Oh, I'm sure you'll hear soon." Finally at nine o'clock the surgeon appeared to say that the operation had been tough but successful and that Jonny was still in the recovery room, as he was having a problem with the pain. "What do you mean, 'a problem with the pain'?" I demanded. It seemed that the epidural had fallen out in the middle of the surgery while his leg was wide open, and that by the time the anaesthesiologist figured out what had happened, Jonny was fully conscious, wracked with pain which they couldn't get back under control for the rest of the operation. While I was absorbing this harrowing news, my son was wheeled past me. I didn't recognize him—he looked utterly deranged.

While part of me felt like a Molotov cocktail ready to explode and take this quiet little surgical unit with me, another part of me was pure *mother,* knowing my kid needed me to be sane and present. It is precisely in these extreme states of being that I have always been most grateful for my practice, for all those hours of sweating my prayers. The innumerable anger dances I'd done over the years had taught me to feel my rage and release it almost in the same breath. I held myself together and dealt with the present crisis. When the time was right, I went out into the snowy night and howled and hurled my rage at the moon, figuring it was not only big enough to absorb me, but divine enough to absolve me.

Mistress is part of us that becomes aware of our feelings and tracks them across our body, bringing enormous vitality and energy to our dance. In a recent workshop I became fascinated with a tall, slender, boyish woman with cropped black hair and cobalt eyes. In her flow she was cruising an old anger. I watched her navigate its course, letting its raw power drive her into a ferocious dance. The *mistress* part of her soul was seducing her, using this anger to fuel the fire of a thousand unborn dances. Her skin was charged with a fearsome light as she danced in the dark of her own heart. Her arms were doing a repetitive movement that very clearly said, "Keep your distance." Her dance was one of smoldering resentment, deep and full.

Arms are the messengers of the heart. They reach out, they pull back, they embrace. When the heart energy isn't free to flow in spontaneous gestures, these thwarted impulses build up in our arms and our hands and inhibit our dance.

A young man in the same room danced without moving his arms. They were totally dead. It broke my heart to see his skinny, fragile frame so weighted down, and I wondered what had happened to him. As he continued to dance I saw an image of him hanging upside down. Later over tea, I shared this vision with him and he spontaneously began convulsing in silent sobs in that awkward way that men who have never cried do. When he was a kid his father dangled him over the toilet with his head in the bowl whenever he expressed anger, threatening to flush him out of existence. We went back in the dance room and I helped him to relive this experience in a dance that ended up being one of those most brilliant anger dances I have ever seen.

People who don't experience the motions of their own hearts don't want anyone else to, either. On the subway, I overhear a perky blonde saying to her companion, "My agent just called, I got a part in the movie! I can't believe it." Her companion answers with a grim look on his face, "Don't." She looks crushed, but obediently swallows her joy. I wish I had a little beeper that I could carry around that would screech "buzz killer" whenever I meet up with one of these freelance downer junkies who don't like it when things look too up for someone else. Be vigilant; they are everywhere.

We usually think of *mistress* energy as the part of us that is sexy and seductive. But what makes us sexy? Being passionately at home in our bodies and honest in our emotions makes us desirable and intriguing. People with rich, rooted emotional lives are magnetic. Vulnerability is disarming to our jaded sensibilities. If we are fascinated by the motions of our own hearts, others will be as well. Until we get in contact with our feelings—our fear, anger, sorrow, joy, and compassion—deep in our bones, we will be unable to communicate them successfully to others and form lasting bonds.

Alive, spontaneous, loving relationships require you to be emotionally receptive not only to your own feelings but to the feelings of others, picking up on their vibrations, reading their bodies, sensing their emotional needs. They also require you to know how to hold your emotional ground and be true to your feelings, even when faced with another who may feel quite differently.

Lori called today. "We have an ailing *mistress* in the house," she reports. "Rachel arrived on our shores, the ink still fresh on her divorce papers, and moved into our guest room to lick her wounds. We just slip food under the door. Visitors come and go bearing good novels and stories of their own lousy divorces. I know she'll emerge next month like a butterfly from a grief cocoon, flap her damp wings until they dry, and flutter across town to decorate her new home."

Sometimes your heart gets broken, other times you're a heart-breaker. To know the full expanse of the heart, we need to experience both sides. Being hurt is part of being human; there's no way to avoid it without shutting down completely. Instead, use it as an excuse to dance.

Dancing with people is a great way to practice falling in love, besides being perfectly safe sex. Meeting somebody in the beat is very straight-forward; how you move is who you are. The beat strips us bare and leaves us completely vulnerable. We dream about being naked in front of strangers, being totally open and exposed. The truth is when they show up, we reach for the towel. Dancing with people for the first time is like going to a nude beach. Initially you're overwhelmed with self-consciousness, but soon you realize that nobody else is looking at you and you begin to relax and forget about your insecurities.

Personally, I'm a soul-flasher, a beat slut. I'll dance any time, any-where. That's why I crossed the Golden Gate Bridge at 8:00 A.M. on a Saturday—an hour I rarely see—and drove through the city to one of those cheap hotel sites good for conferences and jetlag stopovers that always smell of carpet disinfectant and stale coffee. This conference was called, "AIDS, Medicine and Miracles." Standing on a platform with my dredlocked drummer in the hotel ballroom filled with three hundred souls, most of whom had AIDS, I began my seduction.

The beat moved through the room and, in spite of the hour, the room rocked. The mostly male tribe of outlaw angels gave it their all. Some of these guys had been totally hidden away and the only person they had seen in months was their doctor or caretaker. Others had never expressed their emotions publicly; still others had never ex-pressed them privately. The room was ripe and raw. Dancers were crying, raging, ecstatic. Everybody was real—no phony bullshit here. Then I saw the miracle. He was a strange, skeletal guy who stood out in the ocean of gyrating bodies because he was barely moving. But he *was* moving. A button on his white t-shirt read: "Life is too mysterious. Don't take it so serious."

After the session, he told me he only had a T-cell count of four, so walking didn't come easy, much less dancing. I noticed that while he was talking to me he was flirting with my gorgeous gay assistant. Flirting with a T-cell count of four. There should be an award for that. It certainly puts the rest of us to shame.

Flirting is an art, a dangerous art in these times. We need safe havens to practice it in, to work out our *mistress* skills—skills necessary for lovers of all persuasions.

Greg tells me that he works out his *mistress* like a muscle. He and a friend play a game as they walk down the street. "We look someone in the eye and get them to notice us. We score if they turn around."

For two thousand years the *mistress* has been busy selling Pontiacs and mouthwash. I decided it was time to give her a Welcome Home party. I invited all the participants of a workshop I was teaching called *God, Sex, and the Body* to meet at a neighborhood Italian restaurant dressed as their inner *mistress*. I expected most of them to show up looking like models from the Victoria's Secret catalog, reflecting our culture's image of the *mistress* as a whore-slut-sex-bunny.

This disparaging attitude is evident even in the words for the arts of the *mistress*, which are charged with negative ions. Check Mr. Webster:

Seduce, v.t. (L. *seducere*, to lead apart) To tempt to evil or wrongdoing; to lead astray; to persuade to engage in unlawful sexual intercourse, especially for the first time; to induce to give up chastity.

Flirt, v.i. 1. To jeer or gibe; to throw bantering or sarcastic words; to utter contemptuous language. . . . 3. To play the coquette, to coquet; to make insincere advances; to play at love.

The purpose of this party was to reclaim the true power of these words, to create enough trust, love, and permission for the *mistress* archetype to come out of the closet and show her true colors. I wanted to free our sexuality from all constraints and societal labeling, to short out the brain and rewire our perspective, and most important, to throw gender out the window. I wanted a party where gays, straights, and in-betweens could come together and celebrate the power and beauty of the *mistress* within each one of them. The only task of the evening was to flirt with *everyone.*

Sure enough, there were plenty of bustiers and fishnets. But the *mistress* also broke out of her cultural girdle and expressed her individuality with wild abandon. First to arrive was a burly construction worker dressed as a blushing bride. He was breathtaking. A young dancer came as a dominatrix with a black leather g-string, completely exposing her perfectly formed butt. A shy computer programmer turned up dressed like Jim Morrison in skintight black leather pants and a black cut-velvet shirt opened to his waist. A young actor wore a pale pink dress, his sunbleached hair in two pigtails. A female financial consultant sported a midnight-blue slinky jersey dress that slithered over her every curve. Two poets came as sex kittens in black hot-pants, fishnets, go-go boots, and lace zippered bras. A British theater director wore a 1942 black crepe beaded dress he bought at a garage sale for $15. A masseur breezed in garbed in a gold lamé ball gown, silver sparkled heels, and rhinestone bracelet, his scarlet nails perfectly manicured. My friend Don the chemist unleashed his alter ego Donella on us. She wore a blue taffeta skirt with crinoline underneath and batted her eyelashes all night. Don's girlfriend Casey showed up dressed like an innocent little girl, but felt completely out of sorts and finally had to change into a red leather bra and hip huggers.

The night was filled with extraordinary dances. The bride seduced the dominatrix, the dominatrix tangoed with the actor in the baby-doll dress, the actor did the "swim" with Jim Morrison who rescued the financial consultant from Donella. The circular power of love pulsed through the room.

"Funny, people I had been dancing with for years responded differently to me," said Beth. "I started feeling really attractive, and the more attractive I felt the more in love I was, and the more I put this energy out, the more it came back. There was this beautiful, soft, loving, sexual, heart-energy between me and everybody in the restaurant. I had never gone to this place before. This *mistress* place."

Perhaps that's because it's a place we've been ashamed to explore. The gate to the garden was slammed in our face long ago. Flirting is the key that will unlock the *mistress* space in our hearts.

"I finally got it," Lori said after the party. "The first few times I did this workshop I considered myself a flirt failure. I didn't know how to do it. And now I understand that the reason I had trouble flirting was because I always thought of putting myself out there in a way that just wasn't comfortable for me. I finally realized that flirting is not telling somebody something about yourself, but reflecting something about them."

All relationships are about seeing the Beloved in the other and coaxing it out. They are about maintaining your awareness of yourself while giving your attention to another. They are about connecting heart to heart—building a bridge between body and mind.

TO DO (or NOT TO DO)—*Mistress*

Awareness

One day my right hand kept repeating the same movement. It would wave softly and I would be overcome with sadness. After about the fifteenth time, I had a vision of my son as a little boy. I was waving him good-bye as I left him with his dad, as so many of us fragmented parents had to do. This sorrow inhabited my hand and years later I could still hear the song of my heart breaking.

Meditate on your body parts, your head, shoulders, elbows, hands, spine, hips, knees, and feet, focusing on the emotional energies contained in each part. Gently open your personal Pandora's box, becoming aware of what emotions you have stored and where you've stored them. Say you become aware of anger held in your neck, a dream trapped in your thighs, or a sense of diminishment lodged in your chest. Just be aware of this feeling and allow it to tell you its story. There are many stories; each one is a thread in the tapestry of your life and worthy of your awareness.

Several years ago, during a theater workshop, I was overwhelmed by nausea. I had to go home to bed; I couldn't stand up. The doctor couldn't find anything wrong with me. This state of being lasted for about twenty-four hours. A few days later, my sister called to say that my dad had been diagnosed with terminal lung cancer and given only a few months to live. When I spoke to him, I suddenly realized that the exact day and time of his diagnosis was when I was struck down by nausea. I had experienced his fear in my body; it was an emotional intuition. I remember reading about a mother who leapt out of bed at the moment of her son's death in Vietnam. Sometimes the veil lifts and we know we are all one energy.

Action

Do the rhythm of flowing as fast as you can, riding your edge while staying rooted. Follow your feet and keep them moving, never stopping until you feel you are being moved by a force much bigger than you. If you are aware of a specific feeling, pay attention to it in your dance, allow it to move through your dance.

Put on your red dress. I don't care if you are a man; find a fabulous red dress and dance barefoot alone in a room with the music up real loud. Feel the freedom. Emancipate all the amazing aspects of your feminine soul. It's time for a rebirthday party. Make it real, make it raw, let your body rant and rage, quiver and quake, rock and roll, enjoying the full range of your emotional self. Let it all out.

Then, close your eyes and sit in your own darkness, becoming aware of the light emanating from within you. This inner light is love, an emotional prism reflecting all your facets. It isn't abstract; you can see it, feel it, smell it, taste it, be it. Love is energy; don't hold it back, it's the catalyst for your enlightenment.

Mistress Party

It's time to throw a party for the *mistress* that lives in you and your friends. You'll need alluring invitations that are fun but not threatening. Give permission for your guests to dress wild and let their *mistress* out of the closet to party. Prerecord a fabulous soundtrack of sexy, beat-oriented music. Decorate your house in *mistress* style. Think of sensual, sexual, and erotic, scents, textures, and flavors. Screw a red light bulb into your lamp, drape the furniture with swatches of lace and velvet, arrange bouquets of lilac and other heavily aromatic flowers. Think hot—fireballs, barbecue shrimp; think aphrodisiacs—oysters, chocolate-dipped strawberries. Have extra clothes for those who find themselves in a bind and come with nothing to wear. Serve food that is fun to feed each other. *Dance with everybody* and flirt like mad.

Madonna

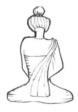

The surest sign that intelligent life exists elsewhere in the universe is that it has never tried to contact us.

Bill Watterson
(Calvin and Hobbes)

In every one of us there is a mysterious Mona Lisa who completes the sacred trinity that defines the feminine soul. *Madonna,* an enigmatic archetype, is the spirit of the feminine mind, a Zen virgin, born anew to every moment. *Madonna* is the part of the soul that receives data, spins it into patterns, weaves them into the web of our higher intelligence, and inspires the necessary actions.

I spend a lot of time in hotel rooms in faraway places. When I'm in a *madonna* mood, I don't turn on the TV, don't worry that I'm missing something. I sit on the bed and listen to the silence, sucking it into my head. Sometimes I track my thoughts and feelings in writing. Most often I light a candle and wait for nothing to happen.

The *madonna* part of us always has a foot in another dimension. It's the mystic within us who throws the I Ching and reads tarot cards, palms, and stars while trying to figure out which point on the enneagram our lover is. It's the wizard part of us that surfs the net and plays Dungeons & Dragons. It's also the contemplative part that chooses to live in ashrams and monasteries, hang out with a fishing rod, or hike the Appalachian Trail.

From Mary Poppins to Mary Richards, *madonna* is all around us. She's a card-carrying member of Greenpeace, voted for Jerry Brown (in fact, may very well be Jerry Brown), and is personally responsible for the six ravens in the Tower of London. Rumi and Michelangelo, Shakespeare and Virginia Woolf, and every character ever inhabited by Audrey Hepburn or Julie Andrews all have big-time *madonna* energy. You do too.

To cultivate *madonna* energy it is wise to practice silence occasionally. I know a nurse who had five kids and yet she practiced silence every Saturday of her grown-up life. Her children often joined her, as did her patients. The power of her *madonna* energy radiated from her and affected every one she came into contact with. It's possible to maintain a commitment to the sacred part of yourself and still be part of the real world.

Johnny Dark is quintessential *madonna* material. Talk about marching to your own drummer—this man is a whole orchestra. He is one of the most brilliant people I know, yet until recently, the most intellectually challenging job he ever held was that of a dog-catcher. He chose this path consciously, to keep his mind free for higher pursuits. For the past forty years he's been writing a never-ending autobiography documenting his life in a series of journals. Nothing goes unnoticed or unconnected—somehow he links the fabulous muffin he ate at 7:30 A.M. on a Wednesday morning to the smile on a Chinese peasant's face. It's all part of the same picture.

Madonna is a spiderwoman spinning tales. Johnny Dark sits in the middle of his web on a park bench in Mill Valley and spins me a story:

"One night a Genie came to a man who lived alone and was sleeping in a bed. The Genie woke the man and said, 'I am a Genie and I can grant you any three wishes you desire.'

"The man, who had made a success in the world and considered himself more clever than the next fellow, sat up in bed and said, 'I have been waiting for just such a moment, and I am ready.' He had previously worked out three wishes and memorized them for just such an eventuality. The first wish was to be omnipotent. The second wish was to be omnipresent. And the third wish was to be omniscient. But because of the hour and the terrible presence of the Genie, the man could not remember exactly how to word the wishes. He was a writer and tended to order his thoughts by writing them down. As he fumbled around by the side of his bed he muttered, 'I wish I had a little pad to write on.' And instantly he held a little pad in his hand.

"He had used up one of his precious wishes. Now he would have to choose among them and eliminate one. At first he thought he'd eliminate omniscience because he wasn't exactly sure what it meant and thought that what he didn't know couldn't hurt him. But he was so slow in making up his mind that the Genie kept rumbling with impatience that he should hurry and come to a decision. Suddenly, the man in a fit of irritation turned and snapped at the Genie, 'I wish you'd stop pressuring me. I can't think when I'm rushed.' And with that the Genie stopped pressuring him.

"Now the man had one wish left and when he realized what he had lost by his carelessness, he was plunged into remorse, regret, and self-pity. But perhaps if he could pick the one correct wish from all three, he might make up for everything in the end. Yet try as he might he could not dare himself to make the final and irrevocable choice. 'I wish I could make up my mind,' he moaned. In a flash, the Genie was gone and the man was left with his mind made up and a small notebook in his hand."

I grew up in libraries, read under the covers at night with a flashlight, and to this day can't pass a bookstore without at least yearning to go in. I've drunk goat's milk in the alps with Heidi, fell passionately in love with Heathcliff, had breakfast in bed with Hemingway in a myriad of European pensiones, socialized with Clarissa Dalloway, been kissed on the neck by Lestat, gone on the road with Kerouac. When we read a book, the *madonna* part of us flows out of our corporeal beings into infinite worlds.

Separated from her soul sisters, she's at worst a mere head-tripper. Over a latte in the East Village, Josie tells me, "When my *madonna* isn't rooted in that deep place of *mother*, that heartful place of *mistress*, she comes out bitchy and gossipy. I sometimes think of Sophia, the goddess of wisdom, as the *madonna*, but when she gets disconnected, she's just an ego trip. I've spent a lot of time hanging out in this unenlightened state of being. It's a part of me that has gotten me into trouble with drugs. *Madonna* can be the temptress who will rationalize anything, who tries to drown out the voice of *mother*, the part of me that cares about my recovery."

I'm riding in a chairlift with a rock n' roll Taoist ski teacher. Skiers float through the powder beneath us as snow falls from the trees. It feels as if we're ascending directly into the sky; the valley below lies receptive and serene, the wind dances across our faces. "This is dazzling!" I gush. My companion suprises me with his response. "I've only recently opened my eyes, to see the beauty around me. I'm sad to say, as many places as I've been, I've rarely seen the light. The top of Mount Sinai and all I saw was a big rock that took me four hours to climb. A spectacular Buddhist temple in Japan and all I saw was an old monastery. At sixteen years old I watched the sun rise from the top of a pyramid in Egypt and all I felt was cold."

Jaded and disconnected from *madonna*-mind, we lose our sense of awe and wonder. *Flowing* has taught me to slow down and pay attention to the drift of energy in and around me. In this state of being the mountain, the trees, the ravens, and the rocks each have a voice that speaks to my true mind, the one below my chattering thoughts.

Where better to retrieve our innocence, that state of direct experience of life, than in nature where time is circular and the laws of rhythm prevail? My father was a *madonna* in his garden. Every day he praised God as he weeded his tomatoes. Gardening was his prayer, his spiritual survival, and the vegetable patch was his altar of choice. That's probably why his last cocktail on earth was wheatgrass. My son keeps an altar in his room. Medicine Buddha watches over it from his place on the wall. A beaded eagle feather, a bear rattle, shells, jade; pictures of the Dalai Lama, Osho, wolves, ravens, his family, the ocean, and the mountains—each object has its place on the royal blue cashmere cloth. My friend Rosie practices tantric sex outdoors. Her body is her altar, sex is her communion, nature is her temple.

We need reminders, rituals to feed our sacred hunger, ways to devote ourselves to the divine spirit within us. Whatever our chosen practice, we need to do it simply for the sake of doing it, not for any outside reward. The point is to find a way into the purity of mind that is our Buddha nature.

Drum circles are a wondrous way to empty the mind. I remember one I did in Taos, New Mexico, with a musician who was particularly tuned into the spirit of his instruments. He stood in his green shirt and blew a conch in each of the four directions. He lit sage smudge in a brown clay pot and waved the smoke around our bodies with his hand like a feather. He placed all his instruments on a red prayer rug—an eagle drum, a thunderdrum, an assortment of rattles and whistles—and introduced each of them by telling us of its ancestors. He sprinkled water on the instruments in honor of their rainforest roots and told each of us to pick one. As he began to drum a simple pattern, we joined in. His voice was trippy—he sang above the beat, an old song bent into shape by timeless repetitions. Then he stopped playing the drum and in the silence began to play stones with sticks. We all circled him like a crescent moon. He put down his sticks, touched his hands to the earth and then raised them to heaven.

During a *Waves* workshop I was teaching in Hawaii I decided to do a ritual on the Heiau, a sacred spot where hula was born on the north shore of Kauai, past Hanalei Bay—on the edge of the world as we know it. Normally I don't like to do rituals in public places, but in paradise how could we not?

We walked to the top of the Heiau in silence. Once there it is customary to find a rock and wrap it in a tea leaf and place it on the altar as an offering. The altar has been carved by nature in the cliffs of the Nepali Coast. People leave dried and fresh leis as well as jewelry and other precious objects in honor of the gods who protect this sacred site. On this day I noticed a tiny rose quartz elephant.

After placing our offerings we stood in a circle on the grassy flat space in front of the altar contemplating the magnificence of our surroundings. I invited each person to go into the center of the circle and create a spontaneous prayer. Some spoke, some danced, some sang.

As we were doing our ritual, three burly, beer-guzzling guys came up and sat down on a rock behind us and, in the name of Jesus, began making fun of everything we did. So much for brotherly love! At first we managed to ignore them but as their language escalated I could feel a wave of anxiety building in the group. I knew I had to do something, but what?

Suddenly I turned and walked toward the men on the rock singing: "Jesus loves me this I know / For the Bible tells me so . . ."

It was a *madonna* moment. The whole group turned toward the men and started singing with me like a cherubic choir. The guys on the rock squirmed, struck dumb. Eventually they lobbed their empty beer cans at us and left. We kept singing long after they were gone.

Dan, a shy, sweet engineer who rides a Harley, tells me he feels his *madonna* energy when he does men's groups. "When I'm in a group of thirty men and I walk into the center of the circle and move through my fear of being seen and I'm present and rooted, that's when I feel my *madonna* power. It's a feeling of being full and empty at the same time. I'm not speaking loud, but my words are coming from my belly. I can hear my voice deepen and quiver with the vibrations I'm feeling in my heart."

Madonna is also the source of our intuitive energy. A couple of years before his accident, I visited Jonathan in Kauai. Toward the end of my visit he announced that he felt a calling to go to Oahu. I didn't really want to pick up and leave one of the most luscious places on earth to go to a big city, but I felt compelled to follow his intuition. We left on a Friday night and on Saturday Kauai was devastated by a hurricane. There wasn't a leaf left on the island after those two-hundred-mile-an-hour winds blew through.

Before leaving for a European teaching tour, I went to a psychic I trust for a reading. One of the things she told me was that I was about to take a fall. At the time I just nodded, accepting her oracle as part of my fate. Later, I would be amazed that I hadn't thought about asking her for more details: Would I be hurt? What kind of a fall did she mean? Stumbling on steps and bruising a knee? I'd stumbled more than a few times before and picked myself up and went on with my life. As it turned out, on that trip I did indeed fall, hitting my head on the hard pavement and knocking some sense into it. This fall represented a turning point in my life and my work.

Madonna inspires not only our individual sense of intuition but our tribal instincts—the vibe that connects us to each other and to the world. Every group is like a person with a body, heart, and mind, each with its own distinctive energy. In the feminine *flow* we are receptive to all these vibes which let us know if we're an insider or an outsider.

Underneath it all we are tribal individuals. We seek connection because we need to know we are not alone on this planet. A taxi driver once told me that no one in his African country gets on a bus without greeting every single person on it. It's unthinkable not to do so, not to honor a sense of something larger than a solitary self. We're not kites without strings—each of us is attached to something bigger than ourselves. We're all part of the same web, spun by the same mysterious spiderwoman.

Some people experience ecstatic communion at rock concerts, other people in sports stadiums, still others in church. I find it on the dance floor, where I join a tribe of dancing maniacs, people who move. I may not know the boy I'm boogieing with, but I know that we both derive from a common dancestor with a Dionysian gene. On the dance floor, differences disappear; nothing matters but sweat, surrender, and soul.

So how do you identify your tribe? They're the people who, when you meet them, you feel as if you've known them your whole life. They're the people you can just be yourself with, with whom you can drop your masks. Lori writes to me about her tribe:

> I'll never meet all the members of my tribe
> But I know them.
> Bumping into a nameless New York Jew in a Parisian cafe
> I know the kind of wedding her mother made her dream of,
> Know our voices will snap to the same sarcastic slur.
>
> So it is with my dancing tribe.
> Another nameless dance floor,
> The barest glance says yes we'll partner.
> Falling into effortless spin
> We chat in fluent flow.
> Elbows ask a question of hips
> Then we laugh at the tired old staccato joke.
> Joined by sweat and shared longing
> to disappear in the pulse
> to move together in prayer,
> Then we're gone.
> Tribe members are anywhere
> and know each other on sight.

I leave you with one of my favorite *madonna* moments. A young man across from me in a crowded Manhattan restaurant reached for my hand to complete a circle of grace. We were four friends in a très trendy sushi joint poised above our Japanese noodles. To the background of scratchy rock music and chatter/chatter/chatter, we held a circle of silence.

TO DO (or NOT TO DO)—Madonna

Awareness

Track your body parts seeking any attitudes, beliefs, or dogmas you may be harboring unconsciously: my breasts are too small; my thighs too big; I don't have enough hair on my chest; I'm too skinny, not buffed enough; men can't dance together; if you masturbate you'll go blind; women shouldn't dance together; don't look anybody in the eye. What makes your head hang forward, your shoulders slump, your jaw clench, your hips lock? The answers to those questions hold the body and heart hostage, contaminating our consciousness and preventing us from being free, fluid, and open-minded. What shadows haunt your emptiness, your Zen mind?

Sometimes rather than a belief or tired old attitude you may come upon an unexpected intuition. Inside your body, your mind is a crystal ball.

Action

Dance yourself into a fast fluid *flow*. Just when you reach the edge of your balance, the edge of your control, shift into slow gear. Don't stop in your tracks or skid to a halt; rather, without stopping your *flow*, dissolve into slow motion. Go back and forth between fast and slow *flowing*, letting yourself fall and then catching yourself before you hit the ground.

Madonna Party

The last time I hung out with my friend Boris in London, we had dinner with a group of Russian writers. They taught me the art of toasting, truly a *madonna* art. They toasted poets dead and living, rock stars, grandparents, old dogs, heroes, antiheroes, places. Whatever or whomever they toasted they brought to the table.

Gather friends together for a remembrance ritual. Create a tape of "remembrance"-type music; for example, the song "The Living Years" by Mike and the Mechanics or Patti Smith's "The Jackson Song" or Elton John's "Candle in the Wind." Dance for as long as it feels right and then sit together. Pass out small pieces of paper to each person and ask them to write on each piece someone they would like to bring to the gathering, alive or dead. After everyone is finished writing, go around and have people tell the story of who they're bringing to the table and then add that slip of paper to the bowl. At the end, if possible and appropriate, find a way to burn these slips of paper and release the spirit of the person you have invoked. After everyone is done, sit in silence and let the stories sink into the tribal memory.

Chapter Five

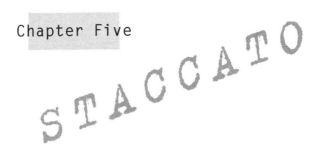

STACCATO

flamenco
kung fu
fire
dog having sex
the crack of the bat
woodpecker
Mick Jagger on stage
kodo drums
funky music
slamming doors
tap dancing
jackhammers
New York Stock Exchange
cutting hair
crunching an apple
cha-cha
red light green light
cracking gum
striking a match
rap music
sushi chef
The Spice Girls
locomotive wheels
Rice Crispies

hiccups
stapler
chopping wood
Charlie Chaplin
Cubism
pinball
Jamie Lee Curtis
fireworks
1812 Overture
karate
metronome
Washington Monument
machine-gun fire
heart pounding
lightning
Whitney Houston's *Step by Step*
 video
Michael Jackson's *Black and
 White* video
Mondrian—*New York Boogie Woogie*
Chinese farmer eating bowl of
 rice
German

I t's Monday morning—the flow is over. I wake to the sound of a box crusher outside my window, followed by the crash and tinkle of hundreds of bottles being thrown into a recycling truck. Just when the shattering dies down, a fire engine blares across Fourteenth Street. It's a block away, but the siren is so loud it may as well be in my living room. As eight o'clock approaches,

I hear a steady parade of heels tapping on the pavement below as a battalion of brisk young professionals march toward the subway. They'll jolt and screech up to Midtown, a phallic fortress of tall buildings often referred to as the groin of the city, where they'll zip up to offices with panoramic views and spend the next twelve hours staring at a computer screen with a phone tucked under their ear and chin.

My natural rhythm happens to be *flowing* but, after twenty years in this hyperactive metropolis, I have definitely internalized *staccato*. "Midtown" Mill Valley is more like the mother's womb. Last time I visited I ordered a tea and watched in amazement while the waitress dreamily walked over to the hot water machine, all the while lost in a conversation with one of the busboys. Her hand rested on the tap as she raptly listened to herself going on and on about the last Dead concert she went to before Jerry died. She was taking *flowing* a little too seriously for me. Don't get me wrong—I, too, loved Jerry Garcia—but I wanted my tea. She seemed to have forgotten all about my order. I sat on the edge of my seat, drumming my fingers on the table, thinking she would be fired if she were in any decent restaurant in New York City. I cooked up all kinds of sarcastic things to say to her that, of course, I would never say. As soon as I realized that part of me was still in Manhattan—or, rather, part of Manhattan was in me—I made myself shift gears. Instead of walking out in a huff, I sat back and took her in like a French movie.

One winter, Robert took me to Jamaica for a bit of *lyrical stillness* to break the intense pressure of big city life. Wandering the beach, taking long naps, enjoying leisurely meals did the trick. By the third day, I was in a very mellow mood. As I stood at the second floor window of our hut, I noticed this young woman wearing a black mini-dress and snapping her gum, clicking down the path in her high heels. I recognized her pace and intensity all too well. Her body screamed Manhattan. Sure enough, just then she called out to her slow-moving companion, "So, Harold, hurry up, my fingernails are growin' here." He stopped dead in his tracks and replied, "Hul-lo—decaf, Shirl."

I'm in a room filled with people dancing *staccato*. It's hot, limbs flicker like flames bursting from bodies. The soul is ablaze, momentarily illuminating the journey. Feet appear to dance on burning embers, hands gesture with righteous fury, heads snap, hearts pump, blood rocks our world.

Just as in *flowing* we connected with our earthiness, in *staccato* we are on fire. Earth is solid and sensual; fire ignites and consumes. It is yang, it is passion and it awakens these energies within us. Heat spreads throughout the body, fueling the dance with unbounded fervor. In my own dance I actually feel it radiating off my skin. Sometimes I hold my hands up so that my palms are facing each other just to feel it. It's as if God were "Burning Down the House," melting down my armor. Ghosts that have been stored since childhood in my muscles and bones take over my dance. When I was eleven, my father almost died and I held this fear of losing him between my shoulder blades until my mid-twenties. Then, one evening on the deck at Esalen, in a simple *staccato* dance, my body started pleading for his life. My chest was jumping out of my skin and snapping back in repetitive contractions. Afterward, an old mountain man with long stringy hair who had been sitting on a bench watching me said, "Girl, your body done bust into a prayer back there."

Staccato is dancing with your bones, creating all kinds of angles and edges like geometry in motion. Lines erupt out of curves, articulating our separateness, creating walls or breaking them down. *Staccato* batters down the fortress of lies and hardened hurts which surround our true mystery. Memories erupt and dissolve in its heavy backbeat.

Staccato is the rhythm of childhood: short attention spans, running from one activity to another, making best friends, writing on the blue line, testing limits, lining up for recess, memorizing the lines of catechism, learning to walk the tightrope between telling the truth and paying the consequences. In the dance it's easy to see the little kid in the body kicking the can, capturing the flag, hitting the ball, hanging on the monkey bars, swinging on metal hoops, hopping between the cracks. Feelings change in an instant—one minute triumphant, the next, left out; desperate to be liked, scared to be seen, exhilarated, humiliated, pious, pleased, pressured, or curious.

In my thirties, I woke up and found that I had no goals. I felt like a case of arrested development. I was all grown up and still didn't know what I wanted to be. My *staccato* energy was unreliable, at best. So I was fascinated when I first met Robert, a long, lean lawyer; sharp-witted, logical, and ambitious. He was like antimatter to my matter. Where I was completely *flowing,* he was totally *staccato.* He knew exactly what he wanted and he wanted me. When I saw him connect with my son, heart to heart, I knew I had found my soulmate as well.

In the womb, the first sound we hear is the beating of our mother's heart. Her body is our first jukebox, her heart pumps life into our every cell. When we're ready to come out and boogie, it's her *staccato* energy that pushes us into the world. She huffs, she puffs, and she blows us out into our flow.

While *flowing* is about taking in, *staccato* is about letting go of all kinds of things, from fatigue to fury, misery to memories, hatreds to heartbreaks. I had a session with a Jungian analyst who worked with breath and she pointed out to me that my inhale was much longer than my exhale; I took it all in but didn't know how to let it go.

I have a student who is completely bottled up; he lets nothing out. He barely opens his mouth when he speaks. He was so commited to not feeling that I was afraid that his face muscles would atrophy. The first time we worked together privately, I put on some loud, angry rock music and asked him to stand far across the room from me and tell me about his experience in the army, which I knew he had hated. I kept shouting, "What?," making him repeat himself over and over until he learned to project over the music. Using his breath and voice to connect his heart to his body helped release some of his pent-up anger.

Staccato is about not only getting in touch with your energies and passions, but expressing them to others, projecting yourself into the outside world. *Staccato* is about doing, not just being; taking action, not just thinking about it.

> *Cut the shit and do the thing.*
> *Marc Allen*

I have a *flowing* friend who thinks his rhythm is *staccato* because he jumps out of bed in the morning. But as soon as he's up he prays or meditates or reads; he sinks into himself. Another friend who truly is *staccato* jumps out of bed, showers, dresses, and is out of the house in twenty minutes.

I am fascinated by the bartender at one of my favorite restaurants. He's a *staccato* ballet, a graceful robot. He doesn't move from one position to the next, he darts and spins on an invisible edge that only he can see. He dodges the other bartender as if he were dribbling a basketball. He doesn't stoop to get the ice from under the counter, he does a series of sudden sit-squats. He whips the glasses out of the rack, throws the ice into the martini shaker, dumps in the vodka, splashes the vermouth, gives it a brisk shake, spews it into the glasses, sets it down, picks up the money, pivots right, flicks the register, slams the money in, pivots left as his right hand leaps from his side to slick back his hair and his dark eyes dart across the crowd. For a moment he is still, but even his *stillness* is vibrant, poised like an animal ready to pounce. His actions seem driven by an internal beat, by the pulse of his heart.

The archetypes of *staccato* are *father, son,* and *holy spirit,* each of which represents a territory of the masculine soul. *Father* knows your limits—he draws boundaries. He's also protective and responsible, your internal *Father Knows Best. Son* is a renegade, a rebel who pushes the envelope, acts on his passion, and lives out his dreams. *Holy spirit* watches the movie from the back row, a detached witness to your melodramatic tendencies. He's a seeker of truth and student of tantra.

TO DO (or NOT TO DO)—*Staccato*

Focus on your exhale, the sound of it, the force of it. Connect yourself to the thrust of your body as you push out the air. Let your movements be sharp, each one distinct and separate from the next. Think of angles, jagged edges, karate, shadow boxing. Be forceful and linear. Create boundaries. Define yourself. Move as if your body were a huge heart, pumping, beating. Exhale percussively.

Exhale as you release each movement. First exaggerate your moves and when you feel you've got it, drop the effort and keep breathing.

Suggested music:

SONG	ALBUM	COMMENT
"Suma"	Tongues	light
"Bush Beat"	Trance	medium
"Tracks"	Zone Unknown	fast

Father

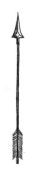

*If there are two courses of
action, you should take the
third.*

Jewish proverb

Another night in the red room at the Magic Shop recording studio. The dumbek player promises to stun me with his beats. My lover rocks in his chair, the engineer swivels, we all listen intently.

For the last ten years I've been sitting on a weird assortment of couches learning how to listen. To do it right, I have to be present and empty. Nothing going on except the beat.

The drummer is doing mathematical hijinks, playing a bell with his toes and two dumbeks with his hands. I like him. He trances me.

A studio is a weird reality; it's like the ultimate room service. Anything you want can be gotten. No effort, just name it and there's someone to run out into the night, or make a call, and sooner rather than later it will arrive. Tacos, Chinese, Evian, Rolling Rock, a Band-Aid, blue movies, you name it. A famous rocker once sent an assistant out to find two art deco lamps. I'm staring at them right now.

We talk about fattening up some of the hits and slipping some beats. Tech talk. The lady with the blue harp arrives. She sits in the dark studio, an avant-garde angel, her fast fingers creating an undertow of feeling between the beats. I've bought four guitars in this lifetime because I've always wanted to play; it hasn't happened yet. Intention is not enough; you have to discipline those fingers.

On the basis of what I hear, I make decisions. Cut this, lift that, bring those notes down. The turquoise and orange clock ticks; in this world, time is money. In a recording session, it's very tempting to just get into the beat and lose myself in the groove, listening to all these talented musicians. But with studio time running $200 an hour, that is not the nature of the game. I have to stay focused and make split-second decisions.

The next drummer is setting up his Taos drum kit. I ask him, "What symbolized the seventies for you?" He answers without blinking, "Miles Davis retired." "Eighties?" "Miles returned." "Nineties?" "Miles recirculated."

Now that's a linear thread I can relate to. The mentor.

Flash forward.

It's the day after the all-night recording session and I need to rev up my engine, so I do my practice to a song on Underworld's new album, *second toughest in the infants*. Today in me, *father* is a techno tart. Heavy beats bring my body back to life long enough for me to ruminate on my life as a masculine being.

Father has been the part of me I have struggled hardest to integrate in this lifetime. It simply doesn't come naturally to me to be linear. I definitely circle the airport on most decisions and process them to death before finally succumbing. Most of what I do know about this part of me I've learned through my work.

In my early teaching days I hardly ever repeated an exercise. I just kept making them up and moving on. "You've done more and documented less than anyone I know," a friend said to me. I thought about this and realized that it might be interesting to slow down the process and go more deeply into things. Instead of just being aware of the patterns of movement that seemed to connect us all, I named them and created specific ways to enter their fields. This was the beginning of the five-rhythm practice. I entered the world of beginnings and endings, lines and boundaries, answers and authority. My *father* began to assert itself.

Father is the masculine consciousness of your body and soul, the active, practical, protective part; the part of you that sets goals, plans for the future, pays bills, and remembers phone numbers; the part of you that functions on the material plane of reality, in the real world as we know it. It's the film director, the management consultant, the traffic cop, the choreographer, the publisher, anyone directing the flow of energy into clear-cut lines. Indeed if you want a whiff of *father* energy check out the maitre d' at your favorite popular restaurant. The other night at Gotham Bar and Grill, I watched Laurie, in a drop-dead little white dress, juggle waiters, tables, busboys, customers, bartenders, checks, and reservations without missing a beat. *Father* dressed as *mistress;* what a delicious combination.

While I was struggling to find my assertive masculine vibe I bought a pair of custom-made cowboy boots. I thought if anything could ground me in my hero mode, the boots would do it.

When I say hero, I'm not talking Bat-Girl or G.I. Jane. I simply mean the part of me that would rescue my own dreams and turn them into my reality. I always liked Sam Shepard's phrase, "cowboy mouth." My *father* has a cowboy mouth, so the boots allowed me to walk my talk into new dimensions. Now I could not only set my alarm and mean it, say no to caffeine, quit smoking, and make to-do-lists, but I could also find the energy to stand up to a business partner who was working me over and tell an abusive boyfriend to go to hell. Dorothy had her red shoes. I had black lizardskin pointed-toe bad-ass cowboy boots.

My son describes his *father* energy as sometimes Gumby, sometimes samurai. I notice that a lot of our *fathers* suffer mood swings. Kathy tells me she is part pilot, part plodder. She goes from instantaneously intuiting directions and destinations on a road trip to deliberating for a half an hour whether to put onions in the salad. I have a friend who bounces between philantrophist and pennypincher without flinching. The world of *father* within us creates some strange characters and most of them don't look anything like Bill Cosby or Dan Rather.

Bill Cosby, Dan Rather, Miles Davis, Arthur Ashe, Martha Graham, Uta Hagen—these are role models, teachers, and mentors, people who have mastered a craft and transmitted the love of it to others. At its best, *father* energy transforms discipline into inspiration.

Sports are in the domain of the *father*. Chasing after balls, catching them, hitting them, throwing them, getting them into holes or between the lines—this is *father* to the max. So is any activity in which you discipline your body according to specific rules and modes of movement, as in skiing, swimming, diving, rock climbing, yoga, or ballet.

After my session at a Body & Soul conference in Boston, a heavyset woman in a bright turquoise t-shirt came up to me excitedly. "It's been a year since I did my first workshop with you," she said. "After that experience, I made this commitment to myself that, come hell or high water, I was going to do these rhythms as a practice three times a week. I took your advice to dance exactly how I felt—tired, frustrated, depressed, horny, or blissed. As you can see, I've lost a hundred pounds." She had lost so much weight, I hadn't recognized her.

Her *father* energy drew that line in the sand, made the commitment, and got her to show up for herself. In the process, it was the change in her relationship to her body, not pills or diets, that brought her freedom. Anybody who has done athletic training or been in a twelve-step program or learned to play the piano has had to call on the deeper teachings of this energy.

I discovered how strong my friend Rosie's *father* is when I was kidding her about going to the gym to get all buffed. "I like to lift weights," she retorted. "I set goals and push myself to achieve them. It feels great to go to the gym and be able to lift five pounds more than the last time I was there. And by the way, did you notice my buns of steel?"

Just as George didn't discover his *mother* energy until his divorce, Eva didn't discover her *father* energy until she was on her own as well. In fact, she can identify the precise moment when it made its appearance.

"I had just driven to Denver after making the difficult decision to leave my twenty-four-year marriage. I left our lakeside home on thirty-five acres for a tiny brick house on a city lot. One day, after a swim at the local sports center, I returned to my car, unlocked the door, got in, and noticed several different-colored electrical wires hanging out of a gaping hole in the dashboard, like the entrails of a dead animal. A few seconds of disbelief, then reality crashed in: my car had been broken into and my stereo stolen, ripped out with a crowbar. Suddenly I realized I was on my own—no one would take care of this for me.

"After dealing with the police, I drove home and fell apart, crying hysterically. I had a 'nun attack' in which I made plans to find a convent, take my vows, and be fed, clothed, and given shelter from this violent, unfair world. Gradually I remembered how much I wanted to be independent and began to gather the strength and balance needed to dance with the experience life brings. I decided to postpone my entry into the convent."

A friend of mine who avoids *staccato* like the plague tells me, "I like to go with the flow and the problem is, the world just doesn't work this way. As I get older, I feel the struggle more profoundly. I spend ninety percent of my energy focused on the present and divide the remaining ten percent between past and future. So, I'm not much of a planner; I'm a very here-and-now kind of guy." Even people who are *flowing* types and we of the "Be Here Now" generation occasionally have to shift into our *father* mode and focus on the future, otherwise we'd never be able to take a vacation, throw a party, or open an I.R.A. Similarly, those with overbearing *father* energy who are constantly thinking about tomorrow or next week or next year have to learn how to downshift and savor the moment.

Many of us are so busy looking outside of ourselves for father figures to impress that we have difficulty hearing our own inner voice of authority. Hopefully the era of gurus and other benevolent dictators is over. Ultimately we have to learn to draw our own lines.

Some of us are afraid of our *staccato* energy and resist boundaries, thinking they will curtail our freedom and restrict our power. But boundaries are not necessarily to hem us in but to keep us on the path. A wind tunnel contains and channels the energy of the wind, increasing its power. A dam controls the flow of water, harnessing its energy. *Father* helps us set boundaries. When I was young and first making my way in the world as a high-school teacher, I refused to sign a year-long teaching contract because I was afraid to limit my choices, I was afraid of commitment. Ironically, I ended up with fewer choices—less money, no benefits, and no job security.

I used to know a photographer who had been putting a slide show of his work together for ten years. Even though a slide show is the ultimate *staccato* kind of project—click, click, click—this man was totally out of touch with his *father* energy. He was incapable of setting limits; he kept adding new slides. Because the show was never finished, he couldn't commit himself to any new projects.

All of us need to know how to operate in a masculine world, whether we like it or not. We don't need to live our lives according to a strict series of five-year plans, just organize them enough so that we can function in the world—meet deadlines, stick to schedules, make decisions. You don't have to sacrifice your feminine nature or your artistic impulses. In fact, if you follow them, you may be surprised to find your life naturally evolving into a more organized, directed pattern.

Under certain circumstances, even if decisiveness is not your natural tendency, you can rise to the occasion by tapping into the reserve of masculine energy hidden deep inside each one of us.

I first discovered this secret strength back in my Big Sur days. Late one night there was a loud knock on my door. I opened it to a red-haired waif of a lady who blurted, "Can I throw up in your toilet?" What could I say? When she was done she plopped herself down on a wicker chair and announced, "Men make me sick." Thus began one of the most amazing relationships I would ever have with a woman.

Susie was the most yin being I have ever known—pure feminine energy. She didn't leave that night or even the next morning but stayed a year and helped take care of my little boy while I worked. In the evenings we would throw the I Ching and argue about men. She drew all these macho types to her, whereas my boyfriends were laid-back, skinny intellectuals—not real men in her estimation. At least we didn't compete.

Susie wouldn't deal with money, which drove me crazy. She even traded Guatemalan cloth when she needed postage stamps. Living with her shifted me right into my *father* pattern. I became protective, took care of all the business, drew the lines, drove the car, paid the bills.

In a strange way, dealing with her money karma was a spiritual awakening for me. It was politically correct not to think about money in those days, so part of me felt like a traitor to the counterculture. But I could never have walked in her shoes—it was frightening to witness someone so entirely reliant on others. How do you trade and barter with Safeway? The good news about leading a penniless existence is you don't have to pay taxes; the bad news is you still die.

Money is the ultimate goal in our culture, one of the languages *father* speaks in our psyches. Too much can leave us drifting and too little can leave us scratching and clawing. Too often we substitute financial interactions for heart-to-heart communications. If we don't have a sense of who we are and what we have to give to the world apart from our riches, we get trapped into thinking that's all people want from us. Or, if our sense of who we are is dependent on our riches and we don't have any, we get trapped into thinking we are worthless.

I was sitting across from a girlfriend in Barneys sharing a massive piece of chocolate cake when she divulged, "I worry that no man is interested in me; they are only interested in my money. So I go for control: I won't let myself have orgasms. I think if I have them, I'll lose control, and if I lose control I'll give away my money."

"Get a grip, girlfriend—or rather, loosen your grip," I replied. "I may have a nun between my legs, but you've got a purse."

During my anorexic period I was obsessed with controlling my intake of food. I wasn't so much afraid of fat as I was afraid of fueling my fire, my passion, my sexuality. I was afraid to follow my heart because of where it wanted to take my body. The more obsessed I became with control, the more I began to assume the shape of the masculine energy—all angles, edges, and bones. This is *father* energy ungrounded in *mother* energy. Control without care.

I read the *Tao Te Ching* to remember my soul and laugh at my ego, to learn how to protect myself in this one-sided world. It says: "Know the masculine but keep to the feminine." The masculine must be grounded in the feminine or we end up being abusive *fathers* to ourselves and each other. *Father* is the part of us meant to build the bridge connecting us to the outside world. A bridge that our feminine selves can dance across, in our own style, in our own time, in the organic rhythms of our own bodies.

TO DO (or NOT TO DO)—*Father*

Awareness

How does the masculine spirit figure in your life, your dreams, and your destiny? Is it overbearing? Dysfunctional? Balanced? You have to be in touch with it in order to know whether your task is to pull it back or set it free. Embodying this energy is primal shit, foundational to your every move.

Think about your self-preservation, how you cover your ass, pay your rent, buy your clothes, make your way in the world. How you handle the practical details of survival. How do you relate to the material world? Is this a strength or a weakness? If it is your weakness, then you probably always find yourself attracted to people who will take care of you.

What's your style of action? Are you decisive? Quick or slow? Thorough? Can you draw the line? Can you articulate what's going on inside of you—what you want, what you need? Do you know how to get it or does it get to you?

Are you driven by ambition? Do you play by the rules? Can you read directions, follow maps, list priorities, make outlines, fill out forms, fix things, break things down? Or do you crack up, fall apart, lose your dignity, or give your power away and blame it on someone else?

Action

Do *staccato* with no music. Connect each move to an exhale and to each exhale add soft, *staccato* sounds, like pah-dah, mo-jo, ho-po. Move and sound like a jazz riff; take on the spirit of Herbie Hancock, Miles Davis, or Bobby McFerrin.

Father Party

Invite your friends for a power lunch and serve high-energy foods. Have fun with this. Dress for success and make sure everyone brings business cards, brochures or their latest work-in-progress. Ask everyone also to bring a to-do list to be presented to the group as performance art. You should be prepared to give a Trumpy Award (you know, The Donald) to the most powerful presenter.

End with a power dance—heavy 4/4 *staccato* driving beat.

Son

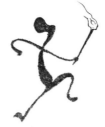

*It's not the same to talk of
bulls as to be in the bullring.*
Spanish proverb

There is a masculine-without-mercy part of your soul, an untamed part that yearns for freedom, the freedom to be the most outrageous person that you can imagine. Eternally pubescent, plugged-in, and passionate, *son* is the wild card, the joker, the fool; a crusader who cannot be domesticated, a piece of your heart buried in the beat of an unsung song. To retrieve this part takes total commitment. It is never safe, rarely sorry, and always willing to be a fool for love.

I think of Isadora Duncan, the son of all *sons*—they threw tomatoes at her in Manhattan but poets fell at her winged feet. She was a prayer wheel spinning in tunics of raw silk. She lived and died outrageously. She broke through the forms of a thousand fathers and created her own dance, one that began in her solar plexus right below her wild heart. Nijinsky leaps across my mind and bumps into Nietzsche climbing the mountain of solitude, words raging.

I feel this spirit every time I find myself in Big Sur. Highway One moves like a snake, a curve in the spine of God, dividing mountain from ocean. Traveling down it, I always feel like a child caught between these two mysterious forces, the towering presence of a dark, brooding *father* and the fathomless depths of a mercurial, moody *mother*. One speaks in silent shapes against the black sky; the other speaks in tongues. Between them, I feel the call of the wild. It's hard to keep my eyes on the road.

Last time I was in Big Sur I went to Sand Dollar Beach for the dawn patrol, that time when surfers paddle out into the ocean to greet the sun. There I was sitting on a rock, Zen mother looking out to sea, squinting to see the black spot that was my son, a 6' 3" manchild riding the waves of the Great Mother.

As my eyes wandered along the surf, I remembered being on this very beach long ago, a young hippie girl doing the nasty with her lover, right here before God and the seagulls. I imagined how a posse of surfer souls from the edge of the world had raced for my womb. It struck me that my wild *son* conceived my wild son, that amazing black dot on the horizon that had just caught a massive wave.

It's a rough gig, hanging between the here-and-now, material reality, definite, direct, get-your-shit-together *father* and the anytime / anywhere, wassup-in-the-void *holy spirit. Son* consciousness is a bridge between those disparate realities, connecting the tangible blood and sweat of *father* to the intangible intelligence and dreams of *holy spirit,* and plugging both of these polarities into the heart.

"His holiness of hip," *son* is the part of Jesus that shouted at the moneymen and roamed the desert for forty days and nights. Siddhartha, Moses, Mohammed, Osho—all were wild men, sons of god, revolutionary spirits. Each of them was a groove monster who moved like a funky bass line, holding together top and bottom, heaven and earth. All of them were taboo breakers.

Son is the kind of guy who tries on women's underwear in department stores just to see the look on the salesperson's face when he asks which dressing room he should use. *Son* is the kind of gal who wears a gray silk dress with fuck-off rock-bitch boots.

Staccato is the spirit of rock 'n' roll and rock 'n' roll is the spirit of the wild *son*. I remember seeing Henry Rollins in Woodstock '94. Naked but for black shorts, "search and destroy" tattooed across his back, he introduced his band with muscles rippling under skin soaked in sweat and sour songs. As he exhaled the rage of a culture, he descended into an underworld of beat and bone, where thrashing, moshing-boy-bumper-cars rolled off each other's edges, mud-men riding the brutal beat. He disappeared into the badlands, hurling words, pushing his voice to the edge. He urged, purged, a primal prayer from beads of sweat—his holy water of choice—anointing his pagan self. Sometimes we need a transfusion; other times we just need to turn on the radio.

In the heart of every one of us resides a drummer in a raunchy rock band, all boy and tuned into the action. This energy moves with us through the life cycles, changing costumes, venues, activities, and modes of expression. Think of Malcom Forbes riding a Harley in his seventies, or Drew Barrymore flashing her tits on the Letterman show. *Son* is the part of me that has been down-and-out and was born to choose; that's stolen from a Safeway, hitchhiked, marched, picketed, protested, eaten fast food, cried at a bullfight, puked at the Oktoberfest, got arrested on the wrong side of the Berlin wall, rabble-roused a thousand crowds to get off their asses and dance their hearts out, bought a Chrome Hearts motorcycle jacket, and never stopped blowing kisses to the man in the moon.

When I was in fifth grade, a friend's mom sometimes drove us to school. It was like riding a bull. A James Dean with boobs, she burned rubber, peeled out, wore a baseball cap and men's shirts, and always had a cigarette hanging out the side of her bright red mouth. Every other word was a swear word. I had never seen a mother like her. Perhaps because she was really a *son*.

Son is a cheeky bastard, as the Brits would say. Not just a rebel, but a trickster who uses his wily ways to subvert the patriarchal authority. Over a glass of cabernet, Robert and I were sitting on the couch as he lamented the fact that he didn't have a wild *son*. And then it hit him that this was the part of him that he had drawn on most as a criminal defense attorney. I made him tell me a war story.

"My client was a college kid trying to pay his tuition by bringing some marijuana up the 'mule' trail from Florida to New York. When he entered New Jersey, he was pulled over by a trooper with an eye for long-haired young men with Florida plates. He ordered him out of the car, searched the car, and found the dope. To justify this, the policeman reported that he smelled the marijuana when he asked for license and registration. The contraband was wrapped in three double-thick Hefty bags, and sealed with duct tape in a carton.

"On the day of the trial, I wrapped three pounds of dead fish the same way and placed the carton under the judge's bench. As he was about to rule against me, I pointed the carton out to him. 'I've been wondering what that was all day,' he said. 'What's that got to do with this case?' I walked over, slashed the carton open, and watched the judge's face change colors faster than a kaleidoscope.

"When he recovered his poise, he ruled the search unconstitutional and released my client. Case closed." The *son* rises!

The wild, catalytic part of us doesn't always ride a Harley. Often in our culture we tend to intellectualize our wildness more powerfully than we can act it out. A friend of mine muses, "I created an image of myself as somebody wild and free. I left Manhattan, moved to Maine, grew my hair, and learned to chop down trees. I became a caricature of the Marlboro Man with a joint in his hand instead of a cigarette. But being out on a limb all the time was tiring and I found myself locked into the image of freedom. I appeared to be a rebel without a pause but in reality I was scared to death of change, scared to death of people, hiding out in the woods."

To be truly wild and free you have to follow your heart, not your head. There's no image of freedom out there. You have to dig deep down inside of yourself to find what works for you.

Look in your heart for a catalyst. Look for the part of you that wants to shake things up, the part of you that takes risks and makes changes. Look for the wild child everyone told to sit down and shut up; the part of you that cannot be hemmed in, that knows lies are dangerous, nice is death, and pretending is just bad acting.

It saddens me to see so many people running from this part of themselves. I understand the threat—it's dangerous territory for anyone who has an investment in a specific self-image, like being the polite one, the do-gooder, the old fart, or even the rebel. "I'm not an angry person," she said, grinding her teeth to stumps. Why protect a self-image that limits and even harms you? Go for the anger and find out what it has to teach you.

Think about the you that likes to experiment. At my last workshop I asked people to let different parts of their body lead the dance. One gorgeous young Brit got so into his hips he inspired the whole room. "My hips just wanted to squirm and thrust. I felt this sound welling up and then a growling roar erupted from my belly. I was overtaken by this totally wild energy, as if I'd become a huge raging hairy beast who just wanted to rampage and roar and *fuck*. I finally broke through all the middle-class training to be such a *nice* boy. It was great!"

In every one of us there is a stripper, a part of us that wants to get down to the bone and peel the culture from our skin with razor-sharp licks of wicked, outspoken tongues. The part of us that doesn't know from sin, that cares about freedom; the part that wants to be a free spirit but maybe can't figure out how. I met a man who lived in a valley on a slanted hill with two rare dogs from China and a house full of women. He was an ebony painter with a scar the shape of Africa on his forehead, partially covered by dreds. The most innocent person I've ever met, he owned a panther and lots of other wild cats. He would go right in their cages, sit down with them, and commune. I asked him how he trained them not to eat him alive. He said he just loved them. I stared at him all night, trying to figure out his secret, as if it might reveal itself on his face. All I saw was wonder. But, isn't that it? The wonder of the wild.

I bumped into Josie a few months after she had done a workshop with me in Manhattan. Back then I had noticed her on the dance floor and observed that she seemed exhilarated when we danced the wild *son,* as if this part of her had been locked away in some forgotten closet. Now we sat down in one of those hip, hot sidewalk cafes in the East Village for a chat. I mentioned my memory of her dance, how beautiful and wild it was, and she said, "Oh, Gabrielle, I'm so afraid of my own wildness! I came so close to having another hit of heroin yesterday. I felt like I was slipping back. It's that wild part of me that doesn't want to give it up. I love this part of me and I don't want to rein it in. One of my greatest fears in recovery is that I'm going to lose the wild *son*. He's brought me to some of the most fantastic places and given me some of the most amazing times of my life and taught me so much because he has pushed me out there over and over again. In the program they say, 'Beware of people, places, and things.' I think of him as the part of me I have to be wary of. I'm having a real hard time finding him and identifying who he is in me now."

"Josie," I sympathized, "your *son* is the one who is seeing you through your recovery. Who do you think stands up in those meetings, tells all those painful stories? It's an act of incredible courage."

I understood that it probably was her ungrounded wild *son* energy that had something to do with her addiction. It reminded me of how my uprooted *father* energy had ruled my existence for longer than I wanted to admit. But I also recognized that it was the wild *son* that was fueling her power to change, and this time it was coming from a sense of care. It takes courage to transform an addiction. You have to admit emotional truth to yourself and be willing to stand up and share it with other people. You have to leave the old behind and strike out into new territories, naked and raw and unprotected. It takes the wildest part of you to commit such an act of freedom.

Son is the part of us that follows our passions and lives our dreams; the extroverted performer who resides in every soul. I was at Chelsea Piers at one o'clock in the morning, all bundled up in layers, for a rehearsal of a one-man ice-skating performance piece called *Freezer Burn*. During a break we were sitting in sub-zero temperatures discussing Greg's entrance for one of his characters. "You blow my mind on the ice—you're pure wild *son*," I said.

"Yeah, he's the star of the show. He does double jumps on ice, back flips and back handsprings. He dances on the edge. When I was in high school I always felt like a nerd because I didn't do sports. Then I realized, so what if I don't run across fields chasing fucking balls? I *have* balls."

Son is the part of the soul that is emotionally expressive, the part of you that will tell the truth at all costs. In the *feminine* mode we are aware of our feelings, tracking them through the body, being receptive to the messages they bear. In the *masculine* mode, we communicate those feelings, risk offering them, reach out through them, and use them to connect with other people's hearts and minds. This part of us knows it is holy work to bare our souls, speak our minds, and follow our hearts into the wilderness of relationship, where very often we find ourselves dancing in the dark.

This wild, masculine, prince-of-tides part of us seeks ecstasy. It desires nothing less than complete possession by a surreal self that can't be boxed or packaged or sold. *Son* is the part of us that goes on a hero's journey to grab a grail or slay a dragon; it is the man in the mirror committed to shattering all fixed images.

Son lives on the edge of the unpredictable, making us interesting. Embodying the energy of the wild card throws the game in your favor. What is required is a willingness to be passionate and involved, intimate and down-to-earth, vulnerable and yet bigger than life when it's required. Balance is basic. Too much *son* energy is threatening, too little is boring, like a red hot chili pepper.

TO DO (or NOT TO DO)—*Son*

Awareness

Do you know your psychic stuntman, the magic part of you committed to off-the-beaten paths, detours, through-lines on neon highways? Do you run after balls or ride boards and wheels of all persuasions? Do you have trouble sitting still?

Have you ever made up your own words to the Pledge of Allegiance? Rented blue movies? Made love in a tree—or to the tree, for that matter—in the airplane bathroom, in the back of the bus, in a phone booth in Frankfurt, or on a straightback chair? Crashed walls, pushed boundaries, lifted bans? Pierced or tattooed something? Worn black lipstick or crucifixes, dyed your hair orange? Are you unable to resist the call of the wild?

Action

Close your eyes and get in touch with your anger. Feel it rise, from your feet into and out of your mouth, like a dark thunder cloud. Experience the energy of your anger rather than your intellectualization of it. Move like lightning. Connect this raw energy to your *staccato* dance and do a very angry, stylized dance. Do this a zillion times until it's art, not therapy; till it has no past and is pure, raw, unadulterated presence. Do it; don't dump it.

Son Party

Go through your music collection and pick out the songs that really represents the wild *son*—his beat, his thoughts, his freedom-fighting, funky, feisty fabulousness—and put them all together on one tape or prepare to spin them live. Invite your friends to a wild *son* party and dj the night away, calling this spirit into the space and the space of this spirit into the body. Be a shaman for a few hours.

Holy Spirit

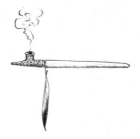

In each of us there is a *holy spirit,* the part of us that actively seeks an answer, a meaning, a purpose to life. It's the part of us that would trek in the Himalayas, become a Buddhist, take a philosophy of religion course, or study tai chi. The part of us that prays, does community service, marches on Washington, becomes a master of something. The part of us that seeks ways to explore sacred yearnings.

Holy spirit is the part of Richard Alpert that went to India and changed his name to Ram Dass, the part of Einstein who broke codes, the part of Gandhi who blew worlds apart with his breath, the part of Gregory Bateson who saw how all the patterns connect. *Holy spirit* is the gatekeeper of pure reason, of satori and samadhi and all the exotic places airlines never go.

Even in our most abandoned moments, when we are totally carried away by an activity or an emotion, part of us remains seemingly undisturbed, uninvolved, and detached, and views the event as if it were happening to someone else. Later, that part of us remembers the details and can tell us if we were acting out of ego or instinct. No matter how successfully we might fool others, that part of us knows the truth, is the truth of who we are. *Holy spirit* is the witness.

I was hanging out at Il Bagatto with my friend Bruce eating fabulous fettucini-salmon-vodka when two Rastas came in and sat down at a table across the restaurant from us. Bruce slurped up a noodle and said, "You know, there's a part of me that's fascinated by Rastas. That whole 'Jah provides' concept is so inspiring. In Jamaica I studied this Rasta friend of mine, trying to imitate his incredible serenity. But I lacked something that he had, some kind of faith in the process. It's an irony to Rastas that white boys want to be Rastas. But in their circle, I felt a communion of spirit that I had never experienced. No dogma, no guilt, no Chapter 1, Verse 3. We smoked some 'timeweed' and sat on a dock in Jamaica just looking at the moon together. I saw my own mortality without ego and without fear. I saw how the whole deal works. We come into existence and do what we do. That's it. I started crying. It was so fucking simple. I just shifted from my ego, obsessing about my mortality, to my soul, which looked right through it."

The *holy spirit* sees through everything; it is the witness part of us that has no investment in outcome, even our own. Think about all you've been through: all the people you've known, the situations you've been in, the yearnings you've felt, the obstacles you've faced, the relationships you've had, the places you've traveled, the hurts and humiliations you've suffered. Notice that through all of it—even through the hard parts—there's been a part of you that didn't go up or down, hold on or let go; the part of you that simply was. Deliverance comes when this part wakes up the rest of you.

In gospel tents or ashrams, under Bodhi trees or wherever people gather in the name of God, the part of us—our higher self—that plugs into universal patterns and guardian angels is the *holy spirit*. It is the force that compels us to seek the oneness of our true nature through action and interaction with others. While *madonna* energy is expressed in an awareness of the sacred, the cosmic unity, and the laws of nature, *holy spirit* moves from the personal to the collective, from meditation to prayer, from awareness to action. *Madonna* knows my mind; *holy spirit* speaks it.

It was my *holy spirit* that took me halfway around the world to meet psychic healers in the Philippines. I wanted not only to witness but to experience their power, their presence, their way of praying and heal-ing. In his fifties, a friend of mine had been diagnosed with inoperable cancer in his brain, given three to six months to live, and advised to go home and wrap up his affairs. It just so happened that he had a Filipino cook who told him that in her country there were healers who did not give up on people but cured them with their hands. He and the cook left for the Philippines the next day. He had his operation, came home, and lived another thirty-three years. Ever since hearing this story I felt compelled to go to that part of the world to see for myself and feel for myself those strange and unsettling healing powers.

At a clinic near the city of Baguio, a healer said a prayer to Jesus, went into an instantaneous trance, put his hand in my stomach, and healed an ulcer. I hadn't ever told him that I was having trouble with my stomach. For me this was a miracle; for him it was just a regular day. I asked him how he received his power. He told me that when he was in his teens, living high in the mountains, his sister became very ill and was on the verge of death. A voice spoke to him in a dream and told him exactly what to do with his hands to heal her. He did, and had been healing others ever since. "The hospital was very far away. God was near," he said.

"In my culture, the hospital is near and God is very far away," I answered.

I met many healers on this journey and every one of them was a deeply spiritual person. All of them were into Jesus; none of them were into churches. They functioned like lone wolves on the outskirts of reality as we know it. They considered the body a series of electromagnetic waves and acted accordingly, parting the waves with their hands to eliminate any disturbances.

I know a journalist who went to India in search of a guru—or at least a good story about his search. His quest ended in a remote village where he waited outside a hut for the guru to agree to see him. He waited three days, impatiently. As he was about to leave he was invited inside. The guru said nothing but began rhythmically snapping his fingers. My friend couldn't believe he had waited three days for this, but after struggling with the meaninglessness of it all, figured he might as well join in. After an hour or so of snapping the guru closed his eyes and dismissed him.

He went to the village to meet his friends, feeling ripped off and disappointed. There is no God, at least not in India, he thought, walking along the dusty roads. His friends probed him about his meeting. He told them nothing had happened.

"Nothing?"

"Nothing. All he did was snap his fingers."

"How?"

So he began snapping his fingers in the same pattern as the guru. Villagers stopped what they were doing and joined in, until soon a crowd had formed, all snapping their fingers in the pattern, in the pulse. With huge smiles, the villagers gathered these three strange men into their hearts and into their beat. The world stopped, all boundaries dissolved, and the journalist felt himself disappear into bliss.

Isn't that what we all want? To disappear into bliss, into that oceanic feeling of oneness? Many of us think we have to go to exotic, faraway places to find it, that's it not possible in our American living rooms, much less in our western bodies. But it is there, within each one of us, within our soul. It takes a conscious act of will to reach this feeling.

Years ago I did some teaching at a psychiatric hospital. One of the groups I met with each day was a circle of teens in recovery from various addictions. On the first day I said to them, "You guys must be pretty sensitive." They reeled in shock. Most people called them dumb, so they wanted to know what I meant. "I figure you were really in touch with your suffering to want to turn it off so badly. Then you were smart enough to realize that nothing could turn it off.

"Here we are going to do something about that pain by transforming your suffering into art. You'll learn not to run from it, but to use it to fuel your fire. Take this room, for example. We're going to meet in here every day. In my opinion, it sucks. It smells like an ashtray and looks like a pissoir. Why don't we change it?" They stared at me blankly. "Why don't we transform the room into a place where you feel great hanging out?" And so we decided how we wanted it to be and then went, all twenty-two of us, to a meeting of the women's auxiliary and requested money and supplies, which they gladly provided.

For the next three days, we painted the walls white, hung plants, made a bulletin board for happening events, hung posters, made huge, colorful pillows to sit on, and created an altar of objects that reminded us of our souls. Whatever direction the eye might wander it would land on a symbol of our collective strength and power. When we were finished, we sat down in a circle in this wondrous space and told our stories with amazing grace. In this ordinary act of creating a space, these kids bonded and a community was born.

Community is safe space. Listening to each other's story with total attention is an act of compassion that catalyzes a deep and profound healing in both teller and listener. We need to be seen and heard; in fact, we're starving for this form of attention. Everybody needs essential attention, that is to say, attention directed toward their essential nature.

Thich Nhat Hanh says that community is the next Buddha. I understand what he means every time I sit in a circle. Each person in the circle is a unique and divine dance, a small piece of the universal puzzle. As I stare at the emptiness between us, it strikes me that our best hope for the future lies in dropping the mind and watching it fall.

Whereas the *madonna* part of us recognizes members of our tribe—the people we can dance with, on whatever level, wherever we may meet, often strangers never to be seen again—the *holy spirit* part of us actively seeks a community of like-minded souls with whom to do the holy work of awakening. This work requires a long-term commitment. It often takes place in a specific setting, such as an ashram or a Zen center or a dance studio. A place where we can break down into parts and sense the whole. A place where we can practice being human, being spiritual, being sensitive and stupid and sorry and silly without feeling competitive, self-conscious, or judged. A place to provide a context for your story.

We find community when we finally settle down after all our spiritual wanderings. If you send your roots down and sink into the earthiness of day-to-day life, then one day you will wake up and have a strong trunk with many branches. Community grows out of being and doing together, dealing with mundane details and domestic dramas. It takes time and attention and trust. A community is made up of the people you want to be around when the shit hits the fan. They're the people whom you can just be yourself with, the people you don't need to impress. The people who lift you up and the people who never let you down.

Lori writes to me about her community. "My community is right here in my kitchen. We know in whose garage the spare futon was last seen, share meals and financial disasters, plant gardens, watch our babies grow, and worry ridiculously about the future. We circle in tight around around each other's crises like hot spots on a war map. We admit our feelings and get dirty together. One bottomless pot of soup travels among us during flu time. We love each other, hate each other now and again, politely overlook each others' temporary insanities, indulge a boring vegan Thanksgiving during someone's Buddhist period and buy an extra pound of Peet's Columbian coffee since we are going there anyhow. As we wrinkle together, we laugh more easily at ourselves. Savoring the warm net we continue to weave, knowing that we're at the age when the rare newcomer may slip into the web, but no one will ever fall out."

I teach a workshop called *Mirrors* in which we track the ego in all its guises and identify the difference between the ego and soul. One of the ways we do this is by performing three to five ego characters for the group, such as Ronnie Resent, Sidney Sniper, Patty Pleaser, Gladys Gorge, or Mopey Dick. Each workshop is a community, even though it disperses after only five days. While together, we serve each other, inspire each other, witness each other, and give each other feedback. The wise part of us knows that while we must take responsibility for all of the ego projections reflected in the communal mirror, we may take refuge from them in the womb of the group. The wise part of us seeks out a community because it knows in this space there is nowhere to run.

A community is a well to drink from, a place to nourish our spirits and find the strength we need to ride life's ups and downs. It's also a place to discover what we have to give. Every one of us has something to share, and it's our individual responsibilty to reach out and offer someone who may be struggling a helping hand. Community service is an active prayer. To be complete we need to serve.

I ask every person whom I've trained to teach the five rhythms to do twenty-four hours of community service a year and document their work as an inspiration to others. This year Angela reached out to a group of hearing-impaired kids. She wrote, "In order for the children to understand my communication they all have to look at me, and I have to stop and ensure they can all see me before I give instructions. This has really helped me to focus and has taught me to have more clarity in my work in general." Whatever you give in service you will receive back tenfold.

Holy spirit is the part of us that seeks our highest level and surrenders to it. The monk watches his breath. The writer follows her hand. Skier and mountain become one. Singer and song, mother and child—

just a series of surrenders. Tuning in to this space is pure Zen juice; as fast as you drink it, you want more.

It is the part of us that acknowledges and acts upon our hunger for spirit, an perpetual existential longing that can never be fulfilled. A holy hunger.

> i want
> my blood to speak
> i want
> my bones
> to break white and clean
> with a new language
> poetry to issue from
> the sweat of my palms,
> language that strokes me,
> licks me open,
> that bathes me
> in faith in the unknown
> that shocks me
> awake
> that whispers in my ear
> that breathes the breath of becoming
> that blesses me among women
> that opens the hearts of men
> that brings love to me
> again and again
> as breath is my prayer
> and the word
> is made flesh.
> i know that this shall be.
>
> Jody Levy

TO DO (or NOT TO DO)—*Holy Spirit*

Awareness

The holy spirit is hidden in your life, your movements, your philosophies and your actions. How do you manifest this energy? How do you express your spiritual nature in the world? In your work, your relationships—in your being?

Where do you seek spiritual solace, in science, religion, sex or art? What inspires you to surrender to the mystery? What do you do with your spiritual urges? How do you seek light in your darkest moment, heaven on earth?

Where do you take refuge to connect with the deepest part of yourself, the dense part that is so dark it is light? The kind of light you can't see with open eyes.

Each of us has a personal, often painful story of our relationship to God. *Holy spirit* is the part of us that tunes into another human being, reaches into their depths and goes for something real. This is holy communion.

Write this story.

Action

Hold your breath and move until you can't hold it anymore. Repeat the same movement while breathing and feel the diference. Be aware—in fact, vigilant—of the tendency to hold your breath. As you're dancing, keep tracking this tendency and when you notice you're holding your breath, let it go. It helps to relax your jaw and let your mouth hang slightly open.

Holy Spirit Party

Invite your friends to a party in honor of the *holy spirit* within us. Ask each person to bring a written offering by or about one of the great masters who has touched their soul. Rumi—Osho—Jesus—the Kabbalah—Sufi stories—scriptures—writers. Have each person make enough copies of their offering for each person coming. After each person has presented theirs, bring out a basket with hole punchers, scissors, ribbons, blank paper, crayons, and other art supplies for each person to make their own holy book with cover art and title.

We Have Come Together

We have come together to fall apart
The queen of chaos straddles
   our corpora callosa
Reins of raw silk weaving our wills
   into the corners of the collective mind
There's more to chaos than meets the mind
   dialoguing with demons, goddesses
   and God
Wings lying unconscious at our sides
   rise and shudder
If chaos were only chaos
   we wouldn't be dancing into new skins
   growing new tails
If chaos were only chaos
   we wouldn't sit in the darkness
   of new moons choking back howls
If chaos were only chaos
   this edge would rise up razor sharp
   and take off our heads
Off with our heads!
We'd eat our cake and dance on the crumbs
Oh, God!
If chaos were only chaos
   she'd take her spiked heel
   and pierce our throats
Ripe verbs would do us all night
Words would fly from our lips like birds
   in a formation never seen by humans
If chaos were only chaos
   the words wouldn't matter
   and the poem would always be there
Always be there
Be there
Be there
We have come together here
We have come together
We have come together to fall apart
                              Jewel Mathieson

Chapter Six

CHAOS

Richard Simmons
avalanche
tornado
Lucille Ball
boiling water
roller coaster
bumper cars
Jackson Pollack Painting
Cairo–Mexico City–Manila
blending a smoothie
David Lynch movie
Jerry Lewis

Niagara Falls
Chinese New Year
Ricochet Rabbit
Tasmanian Devil
Jack Lemmon
junkyard
yard sale
popcorn popping
The West Village in NY
Artaud
monkeys
Disney Building

My mind is a dangerous
neighborhood. I try never to
enter alone.

Anne Lamott

It's a scorching August day and I'm drawn to Central Park by the need for a bit of green relief from the relentless, humid heat. The roads are closed to cars and the park is teeming with energy. Skateboarders, bicyclists, and Rollerbladers whiz by at the speed of light in a flash of color, pads, helmets, sweat, and skin. I follow the Rollerbladers past Sheep's Meadow to a strip of pavement that's a piece of hip-hop heaven. The music blares and blends with a motley crew of live drummers I pass on my way up the Promenade. The beats cruise the airwaves, lingering over bodies laying in the sun, dodging frisbees, and flirting with pretty predators looking for Mister Right. A dog zips past me chasing a ball. A black man in white robes stands on a bench reciting *Othello*. Three people stop and listen. I take a pass on Shakespeare and go for the comic with the crowd. He's performing a piece about a realtor with a Puerto Rican accent trying to rent a tiny space in Harlem with no windows. In the distance I hear a Latino rhythm and move in that direction. As I get closer I see a guy and a girl in black spandex shorts throw their bikes down on the grass. There's a twelve-piece band playing and about two hundred folks listening and munching on fried chicken, oblivious of the sweaty young couple in the background, dancing the rhumba in bike helmets and shades.

The rhythms of *flowing* and *staccato* collide and create the rhythm of *chaos*. In fact, *chaos* probably describes most meetings of the feminine and the masculine, whether within our psyches or at the Pravda bar on Lafayette Street. As an energy, *chaos* gets a bad rap in our culture. Often when I'm teaching I feel the room contract with anxiety as we approach this rhythm. *Chaos* implies being out of control, and this makes a lot of people nervous. The word comes from the Greek word "chaos," meaning empty space or abyss. Most of us are afraid of emptiness because we consider it a vacuum, a negative force. In reality it is a positive space, loaded with potential, free of all the strictures and structures of the ordinary world. *Chaos* has many teachings; it is the place where all contraries, such as feminine and masculine, dissolve; where opposites are transcended and unified. In *chaos* it is ordinary to be visionary, which is why it is the realm of art.

Barneys, an upscale Manhattan department store, has devoted its windows to the aftermath of fashion week: what it looks like backstage after the fashion shows. One window depicts the runways and audience section with chairs overturned in the mad rush for the door, programs and business cards blanketing the floor, empty bottles of Evian everywhere. The runways are littered with invitations, name cards, and film canisters. The second window shows backstage: dresses hanging off racks and strewn about the room, a makeup corner where the floor is ankle-deep in Kleenex and Q-Tips, a half-eaten McDonald's burger next to a bottle of Pepto-Bismol, a forgotten cell phone, wig pieces thrown over chairs, a stained pair of Manola Blahnik heels lying on their sides, plastic bags everywhere. It's a cyclone of *chaos,* the shadow side we all know so well—but what an amazing piece of art!

In the unlikely setting of the Broadway Ballroom in the Marriott Marquis, during a conference presented by Omega Institute, nine hundred dancing maniacs and I went into an ecstatic trance together. On stage, we had my sweet husband Robert on toms holding the bottom beat; Cyro Baptista, a wizard of percussion, moving among the deep sounds of the surdo drum, the drone of the berimbau, shakers with their glass beads striking the gourd, the repinique drum with its high pitch, the squeaky guica and every kind of bell—cowbells, sleigh bells, chime bells, ago-go bells; and Sanga of the Valley, Trinidadian warrior, heart of the trio, driving the songs with djembe and bongos. Together they locked into a serious 6/8 tribal rhythm.

The room became a belly of irresistible beats, each one calling to a different part of the body. First the feet locked into Robert's drum, rooting all of us in the same pattern. Then, one by one, the Dionysian spirit called each body to exorcise its personal demons in spontaneous seizures of abandonment. The djembe seared through skin, raising arms like wings, while the shekere shook heads loose from the confines of reason. Our spirits created, destroyed, and released themselves until our bodies were emptied, the gods entered us, and we were liberated.

A lone dancer caught my eye as her body chanted mantras of movement older than time. She was possessed by a shamanic spirit, her eyes half-open as if she were suspended in the space between worlds, her feet locked into the beat, her spine totally released. Throbbing rhythms pounded her flesh in repetitive undulations; she was a snake-woman slithering into teenage boy, into grandmother, into panther, into eagle—soaring into a zone where she became a synthesis of masculine and feminine, neither this nor that, but all of it and then some. As Nietzsche said, "One must have chaos in oneself to be a dancing star."

As *flowing* grounds us in our earthiness and *staccato* unleashes our fire, *chaos* swirls us into a whirl of water. The body is ninety percent water and it is in this rhythm that we begin to move into that fluid space which is our birthright. The *Tao Te Ching* says, "Nothing in the world is as soft and yielding as water. Yet for dissolving the hard and inflexible, nothing can surpass it." We have become hard and inflexible and the rhythm of *chaos* dissolves us into waves.

As the mother of a son who surfs, I'm often in a state of emotional *chaos*. Every day I say a prayer to the Great Mother to bestow her teachings upon him but show him mercy and keep him safe. When I overheard him telling a friend about catching a dangerous, epic wave, part of me wanted to put my hands over my ears while part of me was fascinated. "It started building up in front of me and I knew instinctively I had to either chicken out and bail or stand up and pull in for the ride of my life. Twenty-five feet ahead of me I could see the hole where I would come out. I was deep back in the tube, wrapped in a hurricane of energy, a mass of water, zooming forward inside a vortex of stillness over a shallow reef of sharp coral. One slip and I'd be Hamburger Helper.

"I can be racing down a wave and go to do a maneuver, think one thing is going to happen, and something totally different occurs. It's a surrender to the unknown, but unlike in my dancing, there's a price to pay. If my mind can't let go and do what needs to be done, I get the instant ax. When that happens, Mother Nature says, 'Loosen up and try me again sometime.' Waves are huge and you know you're going to get pummeled, and when you do you have to dive underneath them and just let yourself be swirled, shifted, and torqued. If you fight it, you drown."

During a break in a recent workshop, a woman in her early forties approached me and confessed a difficulty with *chaos*. She told me that the first time she tried to dance to the *chaos* beat she felt stiff and used a lot of effort. This time, a year later, she let her body be as a rag doll and really surrendered. "After about ten minutes my elbows began doing this jabbing motion and suddenly I was saying, 'Get out of my way,' over and over as if some weird chant had possessed me! As I surrendered more and more to this strange litany, pictures of people in my life whom I allow to hold me back began popping into my head. I started crying, but I kept dancing and dancing until all the images had faded and my tears became tears of joy."

Another woman dancing *chaos* in the same workshop had a vision of herself as a little girl who couldn't have fun. In the dance she tried to make herself have fun. I told her this wasn't a good idea. Rather than impose a feeling upon her dance, she should enter into the dance that she was avoiding, the dance of not having fun, and dance it fully, dance through it until it changed. There are no good or bad or better or worse dances; there is only the dance itself.

> *If you wish to drown,*
> *do not torture yourself with*
> *shallow water.*
>
> Bulgarian proverb

Chaos is like deep-sea diving. We plunge down into the ocean of our being and marvel at the images floating around within us, images that stir tremendous feelings. Often these images provoke sadness, for they represent parts of us that have been hidden and denied. Sometimes they take us back to our adolescence when the voices of our desires and dreams were first drowned out by a cacophony of advice and instructions blasting at us from our parents and teachers. This early loss is particularly tragic, as *chaos* is the gateway to the intuitive mind, the part of us that holds the key to our destiny, our purpose, our contribution, our presence, and our individuality.

Chaos is the rhythm of adolescence, which in our culture begins with the onset of puberty at around ten and usually doesn't end till around thirty. Eliezer, a longtime student and friend, has been doing a stint as musical director at a children's theater company in Virginia. I wrote to him recently and asked him how it felt to be in this energy once again. He wrote back, "I am surrounded by raging hormones, teenagers bouncing off the walls, boys showing off karate kicks, girls on fashion parade, a million flirtations, spontaneous wisecracks, and offhanded swaggering remarks—a vortex of silliness. Meanwhile, I'm supposed to be music-directing a show with all of this energy spinning out of control. Rehearsing seems to be the lowest priority on anyone's mind. But the dance of *chaos* is about jumping in and surrendering to these mad currents, moving with them, and helping birth some shape and form from somewhere deep down under. Over and over again, the result feels like a total miracle to me: a truly great performance emerges out of all that *chaos*. For the kids it's a piece of cake; ten minutes later they're off to the Baskin-Robbins to check out the new babe serving up Jamocha Almond Fudge."

I had the stomach flu recently and it put my whole system in *chaos*. Jesus was born two thousand years ago and that put the whole planet in *chaos*. Fall in love and you are in *chaos,* out of control, a terrified slave to your own wild heart. Life is *chaos*. Nature is *chaos. Chaos* is the nature of the universe.

Each rhythm holds specific teachings for us. In *flowing* we learn how to be sensitive to the flow of our unique energy, to follow it and be true to it, and to ground that energy in our bodies and in the body of the Great Mother, earth herself. In *staccato* we learn how to organize our energy, to focus and direct it, to listen to our hearts and honor our need to express our feelings. In *chaos* we learn how to dive below the surface, logical mind to the intuitive mind; how to get in touch with our whims, our impulses, our spontaneous, poetic intelligence, and free them to move through our bodies and hearts.

We try desperately to hold our lives together, to keep everything secure and predictable, but life is none of those things. *Chaos* teaches us how to hang in the unknown and dig it.

Dancing *chaos* grounds the mind in the body and releases everything that blocks you from your intuition. When I first started doing my practice regularly, it opened a vast world of intuitive energy for me. For a while I channeled this into psychic readings. I'd sit down with somebody, close my eyes, and sink into an awareness of my own body which I would extend into theirs. This was *mother* opening her being to another. Then I'd shift into *father,* actively pursuing and organizing the impressions I was sensing. For example, I did a reading on a man and I immediately picked up a kaleidoscope of images of art objects. I had other images to talk about, but the art objects kept intruding. Finally I heard myself say, "You have a lot of art in your life and it's connected to your colon and to a deep fear of letting go." Sure enough, he'd had a colostomy and had been stockpiling Native American art for three decades.

Intuition is chaotic. If you're afraid of *chaos,* it's hard to access your intuition. *Chaos* is the wild mind fully embodied; if you release yourself into it, the world becomes transparent and you can read it like a book.

The rhythm of *chaos* awakens the mind and roots it in the feet. When we dance *chaos,* we use a specific foot pattern that shifts our weight from one side to the other, shifting the mind from one side of the brain to the other. With each step we give permission to our wild mind to take over. Whatever physical or emotional energy is unleashed creates patterns of movement that express our individual style, our soul.

In *chaos* we are rearranged; our minds are released to flow through our heart and body. If you are true to your energy, whatever is within you will also eventually be released: whatever you have collected and held in the shadows of your body, all that you've refused to feel in the shadows of your heart. Whatever has been held down comes up, and each coming up is an offering. *Chaos* teaches us how to let go, how to move in the unknown, how to die and be reborn.

Atma writes to me of her experience dancing *chaos* at a workshop. "I have a vision of a bird trapped in a box that I saw on the Discovery Channel, flying up and down but destined to go nowhere. The poor bird flaps, glides, flaps again. I, too, am flapping, gliding, lost in the air current. I feel trapped like a poor bird, winging it. I flail my arms several times against the conditioning built into my body. All the patterns of my life hover around, viscous and heavy, dragging me down. Just when I feel I'm about to drown, tears come and I cut loose and fly."

Chaos weaves all the feminine and the masculine archetypes together. As I was dancing with a gorgeous café latte drag queen recently, we started out in the *mother* vibe of checking out each others' flow, tuning into each others' energy and riding it to new heights. We shifted into *father* and began testing our boundaries, expanding and contracting the space between us, seeing how close, how far we could get and still be together. On one of those shifts we met head-on in *mistress*, what a flirt he was, we took it to the edge of camp and fell off into a very touching, vulnerable *son* space—the danger zone of being seen, of reaching out of something raw and real. This opened the door for a *madonna* mood and in this vibe I saw something angelic and ancient in his cheekbones, something reverent and resplendent that took my breath away. On the breath of a new beat we caught the vibe of *holy spirit*, where we disappeared in the dance together, not knowing or caring who was leading, who was following, where we were going or how we were going to get there. We blissed into a state of grace.

Chaos is the space where the feminine energies of *mother, mistress, madonna* are united with their masculine counterparts *father, son, holy spirit*. In this alchemical wedding, the *artist, lover,* and *seeker* are born. *Artist* is an integration of *mother* and *father*. Form without substance is a hollow shell; substance without form is an artist's hell. *Lover* is an integration of *mistress* and *son*. To feel without expressing is to be imprisoned; to express without feeling is performance. *Seeker* is an integration of *madonna* and *holy spirit*. To seek the truth you must be innocent; the moment you stop seeking, you lose your innocence.

TO DO (or NOT TO DO)—*Chaos*

Dance like a rag doll. Shift your weight back and forth—left-right, left-right—feeling the bass beat in your feet, relaxing your jaw, neck, and face, letting your head go limp. Feel your breath rushing through you, the pounding of your heart. Shake it all out, let it all go.

Imagine your arms are great flapping wings. Now flap those wings in the beat. Dance wild, abandoned, uninhibited. Don't forget to keep your eyes at least half open and focused on the floor.

```
Suggested music:
```

SONG	ALBUM	COMMENT
"Chaos"	*Initiation*	*light*
"Buffalo Dream"	*Zone Unknown*	*medium*
"Snake"	*Bones*	*heavy*

```
Artist
```

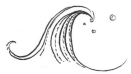

To live a creative life, we must lose our fear of being wrong.

Joseph Chilton Pearce

The *artist* integrates *mother* and *father,* taking all those nebulous, feminine, creative impulses and whipping them into shape, giving them structure, making them manifest. If masculine and feminine energies are out of balance, integration can't take place, resulting in an artistic crisis.

Once I worked on a song for a year, then threw the whole thing out. From the get-go I didn't like the tracks that were being recorded, but I complained in a very teeny voice that nobody seemed to hear. I kept telling myself that whatever came next was going to make it all better. Meanwhile, more tracks were laid down, more money spent. When the song was finally done and after an eight-hour mix, sitting on a torn leather couch as we were about to push the record button, I realized that I really hated this song and nothing was going to make it better. "I can't stand it and I want to erase it," I said. "And I know just what I want to do instead." Finally, the voice of authority I had been seeking for a year! When it finally emerged and combined with a new burst of creativity, I was able to compose, record, and mix a new song in ten hours. Now called "Silver Desert Cafe," it's one of my favorites.

A friend of mine put together a photo show. The design of the show was fabulous—his photographic technique was extraordinary, the printing was exquisite, and the framing was inspired. But the pictures sucked. They had no life, no energy, no passion, no substance. It's as if the pictures were just an excuse to exhibit his talent for form.

It is just as possible to be all form and no substance as it is to be all substance and no form. I had abundant creative vision but I didn't know how to communicate and channel it, how to make the music happen the way I wanted it to. My friend, on the other hand, should have been framing someone else's photos and designing other people's exhibits. Some people get stuck flowing around in their creative brilliance and never figure out how to offer it to the world; other people spend so much time trying to appear creative—wearing black, smoking cloves, hanging out in the right cafes—that they have no juice left to actually create anything.

I met a woman who fancies herself a writer. She's bought every writing manual on the market, certain that one of them contains the secret that will transform her into the next Danielle Steele. She reads and reads and reads, attends lectures about writing, equips herself with Windows 95 and can't wait to upgrade to Windows 97. But she doesn't write. Same goes for the aspiring dancer who buys the leotards and leg warmers, jazz shoes and dance bags, but never goes to class. All package, no product.

When the masculine and feminine are in balance they result in pure and magnificent *chaos*. My friends Martha and Zeet are the perfect example—both artists, they longed to manifest a shared vision, so they bought an abandoned luncheonette and turned it into a wonderfully strange and eclectic restaurant. Inside the intimate, forty-seat dining room everything undulates and reflects, embodying a feminine aesthetic of subtle continuous motion. Candles flicker mysteriously on each table and fans whirl languidly overhead. The music is an intriguing mix of seductive crooners and rolling salsa. Everywhere you look there is something to feed the senses—the flowers, the food and especially, the decor.

Every aspect of the decor has been recycled, bestowing a regenerative, almost organic sense to these inanimate objects. All the light fixtures, for example, were created from the old luncheonette glassware. In two front booths hang chandeliers reinvented as "sugarliers" fashioned from the vintage sugar shakers. A candelabra, or "caffeinalabra," made from cups and saucers, sits on the corner counter looking very "Addams Family." The counter is tiled in a mosaic made up of broken dishes, which they saved for years. Whenever a dish breaks in the restaurant it becomes part of the mosaic. As customers apologize for their clumsiness, Martha assures them, "Don't worry, now you're part of the art!"

By contrast, the kitchen is pure *staccato*. The space is brightly lit, organized in lines and rows that inspire a sense of order and control. Precisely defined actions take place here—chopping, slicing, mixing, measuring. Flip the fish, stack the plates, ring the bell, whisk away the finished dish, and serve piping hot. All good chefs are really dancers, with meticulous footwork grounded in metronomic timing.

> *Any smoothly functioning*
> *technology will have the*
> *appearance of magic.*
> Arthur C. Clarke

When the feminine flow of the dining room meets the masculine pulse of the kitchen, diners experience the true energy of creative *chaos*. "It never fails," Martha tells me. "Twenty people show up right at eight o'clock without a reservation. Getting them all seated is merely the first crisis. Everyone's got their own quirks and special requests. I have to pay attention every second." Some places feature art, Bistro Zeeto *is* art.

Art is all around us and we are all artists. You may not be Picasso, but there's a force within you which drives you to create art. The spirit of magic and creativity you bring to everything you do inspires what I call "everyday art." Life is full of raw material—whether you work at the local bakery or in a corporate office, the level of awareness, attention, and inspiration you bring to your job can transform it to art.

Think of your environment as the excuse to be creative. My house is not my house without flowers. I keep a vase of daisies and orchids on the butcher-block table where I can admire them while I eat my sourdough toast and sip tea. In the soul of the flower, I see the sweet embrace of feminine and masculine, *mother* and *father*, substance and form. Its vibrant life force is always turned toward the light, reaching out from within its fragile stem, through its tiny blossoms, to merge with all and everything.

The space we inhabit speaks volumes about us. Robert used to use a darkroom in a loft around the corner from us. One day I went there to meet him and when the owner opened the door I gasped in absolute horror. There were huge stacks of stuff everywhere—he had never thrown out a film canister, a magazine, a jar, or a newspaper. There was no room to breathe in this space; it was a monument to this man's past and a sign of how suffocated he was by it.

Making a meal can be art. My husband cooks the best rice this side of the Mississippi. Every move he makes is carefully choreographed. He stoops over the kitchen counter to make sure he's at eye level with the cup when he measures the water. He minces the garlic very finely and chops the onions all the same size so they'll cook evenly. He delicately drizzles the oil in the pan, adds the garlic first to make sure it's thoroughly cooked, then the onions, and at the precisely right moment pours in a cup of rice. He stirs and mixes and agitates and turns over the rice so that each kernel gets lightly coated with the olive oil, which has by now been infused with the flavor of garlic and onions. He adds the water and cooks the rice for exactly eighteen minutes. I've even seen him use a stopwatch. Finally, he sprinkles in tiny stir-fried vegetables for color. This simple creative act makes him profoundly happy.

Over the years I have
learned what's important in a
dress is the woman who's
wearing it.

                    Coco Chanel

Getting dressed is definitely an art. I dated a music critic once who chose to wear a uniform. All he kept in his closet were five of the exact same black suits, five identical black shirts, and two pair of black lace-up shoes. By contrast, my friend Martha has closets, baskets, and boxes full of clothes. In the twenty years that I have known her, I've never seen her wear exactly the same thing twice. Her lacy, layered style is inimitable. Every detail of her outfit is part of her gestalt. When we dress thoughtfully and don't just throw any old thing on, putting together a "look" can be one of the most creative acts of our day.

I had a hairdresser in the eighties who used to change her image completely every two or three months. It was amazing; there were times I hardly recognized her. Sometimes she'd have short red hair, other times curly black hair or asymmetrical pink hair. Even though you may not be a hairdresser, there's nothing stopping you from using your body as a canvas and turning yourself into art. It's an act of courage to reinvent yourself, a true way to express the wonderful variety of archetypes that are you.

Dostoyevski wrote, "Taking a new step, uttering a new word is what people fear most." And yet, what could be more exhilarating than dancing on your own edge—leaping into the dark fueled purely by faith in your own potential to become living art? When we take the plunge, we allow our instincts and impulses to flow through us uncensored until we're reeling like a divine dervish. Think of Robin Williams on a roll, Sam Shepard on a rant, or Patti Smith on a wave. Each rides the energy of their own unique spirit.

Words are the great and often wasted medium of everyday art. Our conversations could be art if we didn't spend so much time whining about what turns us off instead of talking about what turns us on.

Every experience provides an opportunity to create a new way of describing what's going on inside and around us. My daily chats with the cashier in my corner deli, for example, have turned into Spanish lessons. I can now name every fruit, vegetable, and beverage available south of the border and am secure in the knowledge that I will never starve in a Latin American country.

Johnny Dark, the storyteller I mentioned earlier, is creating his epic autobiography by stringing together snippets of conversation the rest of the world would consider ordinary. The man is in love with life. "You're probably wondering how I got started on this project," he said to me one day on the phone. I admitted that I had, so he explained. "It began to bother me that so many people I knew were embarking on these intense spiritual quests, taking off for India or regressing into past lives. It's crystal clear to me that everything that they're looking for and wishing for is taking place right now, right where we're standing. Life is so fantastic and miraculous. It blows me away that people don't see it, don't recognize that all their wishes are being granted. I wanted to describe ordinary events in a way that would turn people on to the miracles all around them. Everytime I look at a Van Gogh painting I realize, wow, the world really is filled with color. Nothing drives me crazier than overhearing someone say, 'Been there, done that.' For me life is exactly the opposite—five minutes later you need to be there and do it again. That expression brings everything to a dead end, where movement, change, and the unexpected are what makes life worth living."

> *Sacred cows make the best*
> *hamburger.*
>
> Mark Twain

One evening we had dinner together in a rather loud trendy restaurant. The waiter rattled off the desserts with especial aplomb. "Do you think you could do that again?" Johnny asked. The waiter grinned. "Yeah, sure." And this time Johnny taped him. That evening he tran-

scribed the tape and pasted it into volume 17. Recently he decided to
call up everyone who had played a part in his life story—the first guy he
ever worked with as a lifeguard; the notorious blond poetess with a
white German Shepherd with whom he traveled in a sky-blue VW van;
his roommate who became a movie star; the single mother he lived
with in Tangiers; her now grown-up son who became a news reporter
and a heroin addict; the cousin who owns a music store—to find out
what they had been doing with their lives. Some of them were really
taken aback, while others poured forth. That's volume 18.

Art doesn't have to be big and scary or angst-inspired. Bruce
thought that to be an artist he had to abuse himself and that true art
was only born out of suffering. "I thought I had to be in pain to write
music. Now I'm trying to feel physically good before I create and what
I'm creating is more wholesome because I am." If you think of art as
the way you approach the ordinary details of your mundane existence
instead of as something that hangs in a museum, you can free yourself
of inhibitions that have prevented you from expressing your creativity.
Cut off from the *artist* within us, our soul withers and fades, for art is
what keeps us vibrant. It is the language of the soul.

> *Every child is an artist. The*
> *problem is how to remain an*
> *artist once he grows up.*
> Pablo Picasso

And the soul understands that true art is catalyzed in the wild, unpredictable rhythm of *chaos.* We think we're supposed to know what
we're doing; on the contrary, as artists, our offering to the world is our
unique perspective on the unknown. Art that doesn't come from *chaos,*
from the place where everything is happening at the same time and all
our inhibitions are released, ends up being overintellectualized, uno-
riginal, and boring.

I've never met *anybody* who wasn't an artist. It would be as unthinkable as meeting somebody who didn't have a soul. In certain people

you have to dig a little to find it, but inevitably some spark of genius will fly in your face and expose their artistic self in a flash. It could happen in the middle of a dance; or maybe when you're sitting around singing songs from the fifties, someone you didn't know could sing starts scatting like a bird. In some people this genius is so highly developed that the rest of us can't help but stop and watch or listen to them. I call these people super-artists, those among us who are utterly possessed by the creative spirit. They inspire us, charge our batteries. But that doesn't mean that the rest of us have nothing to offer. Indeed, it is only by immersing ourselves in the creative process that we can truly appreciate the dedication, craft, and vision involved in mastery—important qualities in this culture of fast food, quick fixes, pirates, and clones.

I can make a dancer out of anybody because I know that deep down everyone is one, and my knowledge is more powerful than their resistance. Anyone who can walk can dance. Anyone who can talk can write. Anyone who can breathe can sing. But it does take *doing*.

In my early twenties, I hung out with a group of Ethiopian students in San Francisco. Every Sunday we would go to the park and play ball, then sit around and talk and have a picnic. On the way to and from the park, they were always singing—sometimes the women would sing and the men would answer, other times they'd all sing these delicious harmonies. None of them were "singers"; for them singing was a way of life, of communication, of spreading the good vibes. They had songs for every occasion. They were the most joyous people I have ever known.

When you finally commit yourself completely to a creative act, knots inside you will loosen. I noticed in a workshop last summer that Susannah's voice had changed completely; it seemed lighter, more lyrical. I knew she had been exploring her singing, so I asked her about it. "I always valued my deep voice over my high voice, just as I valued my masculine over my feminine energies. It suddenly dawned on me that I can't disassociate what's going on in my voice from what's going on in my life. My fear of expressing anything light or airy or feminine has kept me from singing soprano which, it turns out, is part of my natural range."

Each of us is an original, with a unique story, a signature dance, and a song that speaks to our soul alone. In his book *The Human Cycle,* Colin Turnbull, the British anthropologist, tells of the Mbuti tribe in Zaire in which a pregnant woman composes a song for her unborn child that will be sung by no other and for no other. She sings this song to the babe in her womb, to the newborn as it is placed on her breast, and forever after when the child needs comforting. In the Mbuti culture you are born with a song.

Your soul will tell you how it wants to express itself; you simply need to shut up and listen to it. Just because your mother is a frustrated ballerina doesn't mean you have to be Barishnikov. You have to open yourself up to all possibilities and let your intuition be your guide.

When we first got together, I remember Robert telling me how deeply he wanted to be a writer. As he stood in front of the window overlooking the ocean, a stream of light poured through the venetian blinds. As the light hit his right hand, I saw images of photographs pouring out of it. Suddenly, it clicked. "Rob, you're a photographer!" A few weeks later I bought him a Nikon for his birthday. He picked it up and started taking photos as if he had been doing it all of his life. A few years later he had a show in Soho. Now his pictures hang on our walls, reminding him of inspired moments and inspiring him with visions for the future.

TO DO (or NOT TO DO)—*Artist*

Awareness

The *artist* is born in the alchemical marriage of your feminine and masculine energies. They merge to manifest your unique style, starting with how you move. How do you dance through your day? Are you in your own flow or someone else's? Are you constantly rushing to keep up or dragging your feet? Do you shuffle or skip through the day? Do you improvise, or is it all choreographed?

Become aware of your voice as an instrument. Is your voice embodied? Do you end every sentence with a question? Are you so quiet that nobody hears you or do you use being quiet to lure them in? Have you cultivated the art of louder-than-thou? Do you come with a warning: earplugs required? Do you turn heads in restaurants? What about your family—do they shout, whisper, or not talk at all? Does your voice reside in your belly and resonate with emotion, or is it dry and monotone? Or is it throaty—do you have that rock-n'-roll-rasp, that Marianne-Faithfull-been-there-done-that kind of voice? Listen to the sound of you—it's a song.

Are you aware of how much poetry pours through you every day as you write memos, birthday cards, love letters, shopping and to-do lists, notes to your kids, the babysitter, the dog walker? Maybe you keep a journal. Do you take these opportunities to cultivate your tone of voice, the poetry of your everyday existence?

Every day you act in a series of scenes, taking on different roles with friends, lovers, kids, neighbors, and others on an amazing variety of sets. We perform monologues, dialogues, lectures, arguments, conference calls. We even change costumes, I hope.

The *artist* within us uniqely expresses our dance, our song, our poetry, our performance. Your art is the greatest gift you have to offer, and offering it is the essence of your practice.

Action

Do a *chaos* dance reflecting exactly how you feel today. You might feel agitated or sluggish or animated—whatever you feel, let it inform this *chaos* dance. As you're dancing, be aware of any movements that you keep repeating, any pattern or groove your body keeps doing. Give this impulse your attention—give it everything you have and keep doing it until it dissolves into something else. Sometimes you may tread water in your *chaos*. Relax in the rhythm until another pattern emerges. Then follow it. Practice shifting between pure abandonment to the beat and the specific articulation of a pattern. Let this be an organic, intuitive process, not an intellectual pursuit. Don't impose pattern on your dance. Let them emerge.

Artist Party

This is the party to celebrate the *artist* within. Forget having a discussion group or processing your lost *artist* neurosis—let's go for pure, unadulterated *chaos*. This is a costume party to release your creative genius, so let your wit loose on the invitation. Create a soundtrack that's unpredictable, imaginative, and inspired. You might lace it with dialogues from famous movies, commercial soundbites, or headline news. The party begins the moment a guest arrives. Have them sign in with a fictitious name, take their fingerprint with fingerpaint, line your walls with long rolls of butcher paper for poetry, drawings, collages. Have face and body paints available. Give a Rodman Award for the most outrageous costume.

Lover

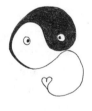

CHOICE
*Blindfolded
I would know
the touch
the taste
the smell of you
among a thousand others
and knowing, choose you.*
Maude Meehan

The *lover* is the offspring of the *mistress* and *son,* of attraction and action. When they connect in us, we can connect with others. When they don't, we're left frustrated and unsatisfied. When *mistress* is disconnected from *son* we become like the romance novelist who can't sustain a loving relationship but spends her days describing them in luscious detail for her readers. What about all the fabulous *mistress* energy inspiring love poems that are never sent? When *son* is disconnected from *mistress* we have casual sex, hot but heartless. On the other hand, when the wildness of *son* has been repressed, we end up doing the same old, same old—no outrageous leaps from the couch to the floor, no stops on the freeway for a quickie in the service station bathroom, no magic.

Kate is a perfect example of how *mistress* and *son* can unite when we least expect it. After a painful breakup, she sat on my couch moaning that her wild *son* was a lost and lonely Pierrot, while her *mistress* was in hiding. I told her not to worry, I had a premonition that her *son* would unveil her *mistress*. Sure enough, I received a letter a couple of months later.

Dearest Gabrielle:

I'm now in Estonia with a company of hearing-impaired and hearing dancers. We are like a troupe of traveling troubadors, communicating in exaggerated signs and symbols—a language silent, yet curiously vital.

I spent my 30th birthday doing improvised street theater in the square dressed in my clown costume, no longer lonely. We looked like those old pictures of commedia dell'arte troupes—or the Marx brothers, depending on your perspective.

Even more amazingly (or "curiouser and curiouser," as Alice said) when I arrived in the square one day the choreographer said, "I've decided to make a piece about Goya's clowns and I'd like you to play Goya's mistress." So I stepped into this dance theater piece as Goya's mistress dressed as a clown. Your prediction came true! I am now both the *mistress* and the *son*. And, I've fallen in love!

When these two energies are in balance, the heart leads and the rest of us follows. I'm not talking about the physical heart, with its mur-

murs and clogged arteries, but the metaphysical heart, the soul of the heart, the part of us that falls in love. Out of fear of exploring our feelings, we tend to act cold-hearted. We have to defrost in order to experience the power of love.

Love has two components: passion and commitment—being fully connected to the desires of your heart in the moment, and being fully present for whatever it is that you're doing or whomever it is that you're with. The bridge between passion and commitment is vulnerability, and it's a hard one to cross.

As chaotic as relationships may seem, they are an essential part of our spiritual evolution, for it is through them that we learn to love. But before we can love anyone else, we must cultivate a passionate relationship to ourselves. This becomes the foundation for all of our friendships, and those friendships, in turn, teach us how to become good lovers. Only when we have mastered the loving arts can we be an inspired soulmate.

Jesus said, "Love thy neighbor as thyself." Unfortunately, that's exactly what we do. Pity our poor neighbor! It's a tragedy that so many of us have ended up clueless when it comes to loving ourselves. Some of us don't think we deserve it, others of us think that we deserve more than anybody else, still others of us feel it but can't act on it. In my younger days, I fell into the first group.

Long ago, I heard myself say "Yes" to a lover who asked me to marry him so as not to hurt his feelings. We were sitting on a flowered couch at sunset in a town called San Jose. He was a beautiful beatnik and I wasn't sure who I was. He wanted to call my parents; I lied and said they were on vacation.

The next day, in front of a room of horrified teenagers, my heart started skipping beats. I was rushed off to the health clinic. After an electrocardiogram and some serious interrogation by the doctor about what was going on in my life at the time, we finally figured out it had something to do with my decision. The kind white-haired doctor told me to go home immediately and tell the young man I wasn't going to marry him. If not, my heart would break. Instead, I broke his. I saw him a week later at a party; he had shaved his head because he'd heard that's what warriors did when they were in mourning.

Somewhere along the line I had been conditioned to sacrifice myself, to say "Yes" when my heart was saying "No." What made me think that some bad-ass, folk-singing guitar player's happiness was more important than my own? I would rather have had a heart attack than disappoint somebody. Somewhere under my skin was buried a young girl in a navy blue uniform who was afraid of being punished; who had no sense of self-worth when compared to others, especially men; and who thought that as long as she pleased other people she'd go to heaven. But since this pleasing bit didn't come naturally to me, I had to swallow a lot of myself to pull it off. I'd like to think that this part of me was simply a product of my time, but I recognize this energy in people of all ages, both men and women.

Years later, alone in my living room, I surrendered to a deep *chaotic* dance that released the lifetime of fear that had led me to betray my heart. In a sweat-soaked leotard and holey black jazz shoes, I slayed the "pleaser" in me. I had unwittingly erected a wall of sorrow between myself and everyone else, my own personal wailing wall. In the dance I tore down the wall, falling on my knees, arms flailing, grabbing secrets from my heart and throwing them right at the center of my huge Huichol painting depicting the shaman's journey. I offered my secrets to the infinite wisdom and crumpled to the floor, body sobbing, shouting "No!" until it became a mantra of power and freedom.

We can't love if we're not willing to experience our fear of all the feelings bottled up in our hearts. One of the tasks of loving is to help each other navigate these dark spaces. If we don't let ourselves experience the magnitude of our own hearts we prevent other people from experiencing theirs. Relationships in which we withhold any part of ourselves are doomed to remain superficial and ultimately unfulfilling. When we persist in this defensiveness, we wake up one day and realize that we have tons of aquaintances, but no real friends.

Friendship is boot camp for love. It's where we batter down the walls we've erected to protect ourselves from emotional betrayal and train ourselves to be open and vulnerable. Friendship is where we learn to track somebody else's emotions and create a safe environment for the other to express themselves. Friendship is where we face the brutal truth: mother lied. We are not the center of the universe.

During a teacher training, one of my students was having a shy attack, feeling isolated and unable to make friends in the group. I gave him a mission to discover at least ten things about ten different people in the next twenty-four hours and report back to me. "Ask them if they're sleeping okay, if they like the food, if they're finding enough alone time. Check out their energy, find out how their doing. Do they miss their kids or their lover? Are they in touch with their feelings or falling apart? Are they obsessing, analyzing, meditating, happy with their roommate? Ask them how they got here; find out where they're going." By the next day, he was completely in the flow of things. "I can't believe it. I always thought that in order to relate to other people I had to talk about myself, to perform. Doing this task I realized that to make friends I simply have to be aware of myself and pay attention to who I am with."

Friendship is the backbone of all our relationships, the blueprint for all other heart-to-heart interactions. We have to help each other fight the impulse to put ourselves and each other into neat little boxes and pigeon holes so we can keep everything predictable, secure, and under control. Rather than diminish each other this way, true friends support each other's wildness and expansiveness and respect each other's unknown, mysterious selves.

Larry was tired of hearing his friends moan about not having lovers so he wrote personal ads for them. Talk about getting by with a little help from our friends!

MEN SEEKING MEN

1962 Hot Rod

(Soul driver.) White sporty coupe w/purring engine, great bumpers, solid brakes. Cruising controlled and horsey powered. Long-term lease or sale only. ISO confident driver who can surrender to the road. No DWI's.

WOMEN SEEKING MEN
Medusa Curls
(I'm less deadly.) Drumming, dancing, SWF delight, 29, 5 6, ISO strapping, funky, clever, physical man who can T.C.B. Like me, be (a) heart-warrior, body-mind-spirit seeker. Never say "should."

Who doesn't long to love? The day after I met Robert, I remember thinking to myself, "Wow, I don't see the end." Before that, I had always envisioned the end of a relationship in the beginning, how it fit into my three-year plan. This time was different, it was real. Falling in love threw me into total *chaos*—I realized that in order to be true to my heart, I'd have to leave my roots, my work, and my friends and move clear across the continent. I knew what I wanted and when I said "Yes," this time I meant it with my whole self. Of course, I did freak out a bit, but Robert was right there for me—he was my best friend.

Loving friends and respecting their individuality is an essential foundation for being lovers. That foundation has to be rock-solid because when sex rears its beautiful head, all walls come crashing down. In the act of sex, we are fully exposed in all of our vulnerability, in all of our *chaos,* and we need to know that we're unconditionally supported in this naked state. As lovers, the stakes are raised, and without a safety net we have a lot further to fall. We have more to give and more to get, and we must offer nothing less than ourselves—body and soul. Jesus said, "Drink me. Eat me." He offered himself as holy communion. And he was the ultimate *lover.*

> *There is nothing safe about*
> *sex. There never will be.*
> *Norman Mailer*

Making love is an art that requires practice. We need to be able to talk about sex openly, do it freely, develop a little expertise. You don't have to be in a Calvin Klein ad to fuel somebody's obsession. *Lovers* help each other feel good about their bodies. We can never be at ease with ourselves or each other if we are uptight about our sexuality. It's one of the most important forces in our lives; we are created out of sex, every cell of us is sexual.

To become a *lover*, we must fall in love with love—lose our heads to our hearts, delve into unmapped, unrehearsed territory, and dispense with whatever macho and romantic illusions we've been force-fed all our lives. One of the greatest of these illusions is that we know something about love. Why don't we just admit it? When it comes to loving we are babes in the woods. So let's just go with the flow, surrender to the *chaos*, and take whatever comes.

Brad was always a straight-and-narrow kind of guy until he blew his whole image by being with three women in one week. Since he had been working the scarcity principle for quite a while, this put him in a state of shock. "My conservative conditioning was freaking. Each woman was so different, each brought out a different me. Joy brought out the wild *son*—sex with her was dangerous, we were crawling the walls. She seduced me hardcore; in the bedroom she had no boundaries and I had never been near this territory before. The very next night Terri Mae brought out my *madonna*, with her candles, incense, and massage. We made love right under a picture of Jesus. And two nights later Georgette gave me a blow job while I was driving my car at sixty miles per hour. I'm telling you, my roommates hated me! But something was turning on inside me that I didn't want to turn off."

Drag my lips across these mouths
drag my hips across this crowd
Curiosity knows no bounds
I'd love to sleep with the whole town.

Tim Booth

The *lover* isn't always convenient and is rarely conservative unless it's imprisoned in dogmas that don't dance, beliefs that don't serve, and theories that bind. In the beginning I believe we need lots of lovers to explore all the aspects of our own. Each one catalyzes new feelings, each one teaches us a lesson, each one opens us a little bit more to our deepest needs and desires.

Sometimes a lover will jolt us into becoming aware of a part of ourselves we didn't know existed. Eva remembers the first time she danced with a woman. "It was during a workshop. I went to give a girlfriend a hug and she started dancing with me real close, body-to-body, like we did in high school, and I got turned on. Becoming aware of this response was the beginning of my healing. It was like falling out of a dream. I had been married for twenty years and had no idea why sex with my husband did not turn me on. I thought that if I tried hard enough, I would learn to respond to him, but I didn't and I blamed myself. I lived in this hell every day and dreaded it every night. By the end of that dance, I realized that before I died I wanted to be with a woman."

The *lover* is the part of us that yearns for sexual ecstasy, and *chaos* is the key to unlocking our erotic potential. Unfortunately, most men and women are clueless when it comes to falling apart in each other's arms. Considering how many women have never had orgasms, it looks like the Good Girl Party is still in power.

It's time for a revolution. I'm not talking about a feminist revolution or a political coup; I'm talking about a revolution in thought. The position of the mind is the most radical position in sex and our heads are still doing it missionary style. It's time to follow our instincts, attractions, and desires and go where they take us with integrity and love. The body has no theories or dogmas, it is simply part of the dance. The body doesn't even make relationships, it just carries them out. Energy makes relationships and a good relationship is going to have a healthy balance of masculine and feminine energies; no matter what kind of bodies they come in. I have a friend who left her husband for another woman with whom she bonded and whom she considers her soulmate. The one time they broke up for a spell they both dated men. When I asked Lori her sexual preference, she stated, "Cardio-sexual."

If we find ourselves attracted to the same sex, it's important to follow these impulses, otherwise we'll spend the rest of our lives stuck in

a state of thwarted ecstasy, our repressed yearning gnawing a hole in
our very soul.

> *Not until the male*
> *becomes female and the*
> *female becomes male shall ye*
> *enter the kingdom of Heaven.*
>
> *Jesus*
> *The Gospel of St. Thomas*

On the last day of a workshop, a young woman in her early thirties
came up to me and whispered in my ear, "Last night I had my first orgasm." She stood there looking like a neon version of Botticelli's *Venus.*
She told me that she and her lover had made love in the woods under
a full moon. "We had never begun in *flowing* before—my boyfriend is a
speedy kind of guy. He usually entered me in a very *staccato* way and
then he'd go immediately into *chaos* and I'd feel left behind. My body
doesn't move that fast. He's a pressure cooker and I'm more of a slow
boil." So right, little sister.

> *This bed is on fire with*
> *passionate love—*
> *the neighbors complained*
> *about the noises above—*
> *but she only comes when*
> *she's on top.*
>
> *Tim Booth*

Of course, orgasms aren't the be-all and end-all. Rather, they're a
means to shattering into a lightness of being that takes us past ourselves, past our lovers, and illuminates the divine emptiness that beck-
ons us into its embrace. The blissed-out, post-coital mind is nothing
but a meditation on loving.

Once you've learned to love yourself, share that love with a friend, and express that love through sex, you're ready to find your soulmate. At this level, love reaches beyond the boundaries of coupledom out to the world at large. Families merge and emerge, tribes grow, communities take root.

As the era of the fragmented family seems to be drawing to a close, perhaps we can gain some perspective on what went wrong. To my mind, part of the problem was that people leapt into marriage without first developing the arts necessary to be a friend, a lover, and a soulmate. Without these skills, marriage—our culture's way of bonding soulmates—is doomed to fail. If it's not about our mutual growth toward god consciousness, toward a commitment to each other's awakening—to the depths rather than the surface—if it's about money or duty or expectation, we'll inevitably end up angry, frustrated, and bored.

> *I think men who have a*
> *pierced ear are better*
> *prepared for marriage.*
> *They've experienced pain*
> *and bought jewelry.*
> Rita Rudner

Sometimes marriages fail because people are so focused on the other they lose sight of themselves; other times, they're so focused on themselves they lose sight of the other. Ideally, we're focused on the energy—the love—that moves between us. Soulmates become an excuse to surrender to the Beloved.

I know two people who truly love each other and yet they can't make their marriage work. He wants a wife who is going to be the center of his world, for whom the relationship will be both her vocation and her avocation. She wants a partner and a lover who is going to cheer her on as she goes out into the bigger world. If either one tries to change to please the other it initiates a cycle of resentment and loathing. They're like Romeo and Juliet, except the forces sabotaging their relationship come from within them. And in the psychic torment that this has created for them, they see no option but to separate.

The real problem is that both have a picture of what their relationship should look like, but it's not the same picture. It's my belief that all pictures are dangerous. When you try to shoehorn your relationship into somebody else's shoe, whether it's *Ozzie and Harriet* or *When Harry Met Sally,* you only end up with blisters and bunions. Relationship is *chaos.* To try to control it is to dishonor its vitality, its individuality, its divine dance.

Lovers love for the sake of loving; they jump heart-first into all situations. A truly passionate loving relationship lives in the moment and embraces *chaos.* While we may make plans for the future, it's wise to remain flexible, leaving room for each of us to change and grow and develop in unpredictable ways. If we don't acknowledge the role of the unknown, our relationship becomes a scripted performance.

Imaginative *lovers* rule. Martha came home from work on her birthday to find her husband dressed as a geisha. He had made her an elaborate tea and while she partook he massaged her tiny feet. Then he put her in a luscious candlelit bubble bath and when she came out, he was in their bed, in a beautiful white dress. "Come and get your birthday present," he smiled ever so slyly.

What holds us back from plunging into the *chaos* of our relationships is our deep-seated fear of intimacy. Most of us are scared to death of the big "I." We need it, we want it, but when we come within spitting distance of it we take off in the opposite direction. We hold on, we hold back, we hold out. We avoid eye contact for fear that it will reveal our confusion. We want the other person to be open, vulnerable, and passionate, to act with integrity, yet we balk at doing the same. Intimacy is not a one-way street—you have to give to get. Our relationships are a measure of what we're willing to give. People are always complaining that nobody loves them, they're all alone. I say, "Love somebody, then. Whatever you want, give it away."

For years I was terrified of commitment and intimacy so I kept myself split. I would either have a deep, passionate, sexual relationship with someone I had nothing in common with or I would be with someone who was intellectually stimulating and loving, but boring in bed. As long as I kept one part of me protected at all times, my body or my head, I was safe.

There is a beauty in overcoming our fear of intimacy, in letting go and allowing ourselves to experience the intensity of *chaos* in all its spontaneous brilliance.

As *lovers,* we ride the wild waves of wine-dark seas on our journey to the heart of the Beloved. This is not a solo odyssey, however. Although it begins with self-discovery, it ends with a release of self into the chaotic cosmos, into the magical mystery that is at the core of each one of us, into the spirit of God.

She calls to the wildman
dancing naked by the shores
of the ocean that she is,
He who speaks with tigers,
whose muscles move with
slow liquid grace.
He who no longer fears
his darkness, or
the stillness of the earth, or
the sometimes suffocating pull
of her relentless rhythms,
gravities and tides,
He who has made his peace
with Kali and the void,
he who no longer needs
to run or hide
from the sweet source of power
calling him from deep
inside.

Jody Levy

TO DO (or NOT TO DO)—*Lover*

Awareness

Make a list of all your lovers from the beginning to now. In case you don't remember their names, brief physical descriptions will do. Are you on the list? What's your frequency of self-lovemaking, or do you roll over in bed and read a self-help book? Just checking. Now look at your list. Based on sheer numbers alone, what does it say to you? If all these lovers were to appear in your bedroom as a Greek chorus, what would be their chant, their lament, their cheer? Study this list and label each person on it by their most prominent archetypes—*mother, mistress, madonna, father, son, holy spirit.* If any embodies them all, put a star next to their name and check your phone book to see if you still have their telephone number. What have you learned from this? Do you tend to attract *fathers* or *madonnas*? Use this same list to imagine how each one of them would categorize you. What role did you play in their lives? The provider, the catalyst, the sex kitten, the heartbreaker? Be poetic; you're an *artist*.

Action

I recommend the "Roth Rhythm Method," whether you are alone or with someone else. First, practice being the *flowing* lover. Put on *flowing* music and create a totally flowing, feminine, sensual, earthy space, however you imagine that to be. Immerse yourself in this rhythm and make it your mission to awaken this rhythm in your lover. Now practice being the *staccato* lover: use funky music; make love in a chair, up against the wall, in the back seat of a car. Practice being the *chaotic* lover. Get animal, down to the basics; make sounds. Make love on the beach, in the woods, to techno-tribal music. Be wild, unpredictable, and totally creative in your approach. Practice being the *lyrical* lover. Be playful, whimsical, magical. Make love to classical music. Practice being the *still* lover. Make love to Tibetan chant music or whatever invokes spirit for you. Try to move as little as possible, to listen to your lovers' body, even if it's the one you're in. Try not to have an orgasm. Focus on your two bodies or your own merging into a timeless, egoless zone.

The Lover Party

The *lover* party is not a pajama party (unless you want it to be), but a writing circle. Hang out with some close friends and entertain and educate each other with your stories. Here are some suggestions for writing topics:

1. Losing your virginity.
2. Your wildest or best sex.
3. Your ultimate sexual fantasy.
4. Jumping gender boundaries in mind or body.
5. A fatal attraction.
6. Your parents' sex life.
7. A time you felt empowered by a lover.
8. A time when you empowered the *lover* in someone else.

Seeker

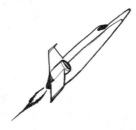

I have been and still am a seeker, but I have ceased to question stars and books; I have begun to listen to the teachings my blood whispers to me.

Herman Hesse

The *seeker* is an integration of *madonna* and *holy spirit*, of innocence and wisdom. The *seeker* is a state of mind, the metaphor of our existence. When we are in our intuitive mind, our *seeker*-mind, we don't need to think. We can just be in the moment, open to experience. From direct experience comes wisdom, which is quite different from knowledge. Knowledge is rooted in external sources and absorbed from the surrounding culture. Wisdom only comes when we empty our minds, free them from the strictures of knowledge.

Seeker is the drive to find order in *chaos,* to seek the underlying patterns and find the internal, eternal, enduring themes and connections that give a sense of meaning to our lives. We have to trust that such patterns exist even though they might be bigger than the individual eye can see. Otherwise we end up drifting through a nihilistic landscape—not a pretty place to be. That trust is a leap of faith. Maybe it's because I'm a dancer, but leaping into the void doesn't scare me. Inside me, *seeker* is faith.

I can't think of a person who doesn't need more faith. Not religious faith, but faith in the process, in who we are and what we're doing, how we got here and where we're going. Too many of us don't trust that there is a bigger picture out there; instead, we anxiously paper the walls of our minds with snapshots of how we think our lives are supposed to be. To experience faith we have to clear away all the clutter until our minds are like tabula rasa. For me, faith happens when my mind is in my feet and I'm not thinking at all.

I was scheduled to give a talk a couple of years ago at St. James Church in Piccadilly Circus. For some strange reason, I brought my drummer, Sanga, along. (I always keep a drummer in the trunk of my car. They come in handy.) He showed up with his djembe looking insecure. I guess all the people sitting in pews unnerved him.

The evening began with a candle ceremony. Two women came up to the altar and each one lit a taper and picked a quality to call forth into the room. I lit the third and picked faith.

Five hundred faces gazed at me expectantly, yet I had no idea what I was going to say. One thing I did know was that faith is the bridge between innocence and wisdom, so I sank into the marble memory of the floor and let myself cross this bridge. My feet knew we were ripe for some *chaos* in this stone-cold church, so I signaled Sanga to begin the beat.

I started whirling in a circle beneath the gilded dome, wishing Sister Mary Alberta could see me now. I coaxed the heads to drop, the shoulders to release, the faces to relax, and the bodies to rise up from the pews and move out into the aisles. For centuries I had wanted to get up off my knees and dance around an altar, to create a litany of limbs in honor of the God within us—the dance inside the dancer, the current inside the flow. I conjured an image of *madonna* doing a tango with *holy spirit*. In this marriage, the *seeker* delivers us to the Beloved as surely as *mother* delivers us to earth.

When it all ended, I talked with Harry, the Australian sound man, and discovered he was a mathemetician by training. "That means we have a lot in common," I said. "We're both possessed by zero."

Zero mind is *seeker* territory, the origin of dreams. Dreams are utter *chaos,* a private screening of the intuitive mind. Dreams are often very wise. For example, when I was in Utah, the night before Jonathan's surgery, I dreamt that Jonny had two huge snakes in his mouth. They curled around his spine and came out his anus. I woke up knowing that he would heal himself.

Before I left for the trip to London in which I ended up in St. James Church, I dreamt I was in a car accident on a coastal road. On my way to London, I stopped in Majorca to spend a week with my friend Lynn. Driving to the airport after a blissful vacation, we rounded a hairpin curve and found ourselves face-to-face with a huge red tour bus. It was either crash into the bus or drive over the cliff. Lynn chose the bus. I thought she made a wise decision.

I arrived in London with internal injuries, a serious concussion, and a very intense teaching schedule. Everyone thought I should cancel—everyone but me. I felt that since I had dreamt the accident, it and all its aftermath were meant to be. I put my faith in this possibility and proceeded to teach, dubbing this tour "The Wounded Healer Rides Again."

I blew my martyr act by acknowledging that I needed an osteopath. I was given a list with ten names, but didn't have a clue how to choose one. So I read the list and closed my eyes and one name stuck in my head. Even though his was the most inconvenient location on the list, I called and made an appointment. I was operating on faith.

My osteopath was a soft-spoken, *madonna* kind of guy who worked in a tiny room, bare but for a table and a replica of a skeleton on the wall. In my fifth session, as he was holding my head, it kept moving to the right. He asked me, "What is your head trying to say?" Without missing a beat, I immediately stated, "Be a Buddhist." Wow! This was news to me. "And how do you feel about that," he almost whispered. "Very sad." And as I lay on the table feeling the intense warmth of his hands radiating into my head, I was overcome by a profound sense of yearning. He probed me about this and I heard myself say, "I've been looking for my teacher for two thousand years." I felt the deep truth in this statement but it had never occurred to me that I harbored such a feeling.

After the session the osteopath invited me to have tea at a little shop nearby. Over Earl Gray and scones with clotted cream, he confided to my utter amazement that he was a Tibetan Buddhist. He then told me the story of how he met his teacher which touched me very deeply. As he spoke I kept seeing images of monks from my dreams—a Tibetan monk in a cowboy hat, an elderly monk running down a steep hill with a child on his back, a fiery young monk addressing a group of people seated on rows of wooden benches. He promised he would ask his teacher to call me when he came to New York in a few months' time.

I returned to Manhattan and got back into the swing of my hectic life and, as my injuries healed, forgot all about my sweet osteopath. One day, several months later, the phone rang and it was his teacher who had just arrived in New York.

We met the next morning for a Japanese breakfast in the Grand Hyatt Hotel. When we were done, I asked him what he would like to do. Would he like to go to Central Park? "A park is just a park," he answered softly. Maybe he'd like to visit one of our great museums. "A museum is just a museum." And then it hit me, "Well then, let's go to Bloomingdale's." He lit up.

For the rest of the morning, we rode the escalators at Bloomingdale's, a monk in crimson and gold and a lady in black, sun and void, shopping for nothing, knowing there is nothing. Occasionally we'd stroll through the floors, looking at clothes and furniture and appliances. We stopped and admired the leather goods; he had a penchant for wallets but no need for one, as he never handled money. It was a weird kind of therapy for me to shop with a monk.

As we walked up Lexington Avenue, I said, "Sometimes my mind is not in my feet and I feel a million miles away from who I am." He told me that he had never felt separated from his feet. It must be a western phenomenon, I thought to myself. But as we walked I sensed he suffered a different kind of longing, an aching to be free, to move like the wind, unfettered by tradition just for a moment. I heard it between his lines as he mentioned to me that in his homeland he can't go for a walk without a few thousand people following him. "But you can leave if you want, can't you?" He laughed. "Oh yes, I am trapped in a golden prison, but I don't want to escape without wisdom." I thought about that word. How many of us truly want wisdom? We want many things but who really wants to be wise?

Last year the Dalai Lama spoke in Manhattan and a woman asked him what he had to say about the fragmented western family. "Be affectionate," he answered with a lovely smile on his face. That is the difference between a Tibetan kid and the lonely boy in the baseball lot on many American streets: the Tibetan soul is nurtured with wisdom, humor, and affection and it shows on their contented faces. Even though they face many of the same demons that all of us face, they are better equipped by their culture. No wonder I dream about Tibetan monks.

I learned a lot of surprising things about that monk during our few hours together, including that we read the same fantasy fiction. Oddly enough, I had been a little embarrassed to admit my Tolkien fetish to him. Now I felt redeemed. I've always believed that fantasy fiction feeds the spirit of my mind, the part of me which remembers the magic, travels with unbelievers, meets talking trees and wizards, moves in an imaginary world. The part of me that reads fantasy novels is the same part of me that knows my life is fiction—no hard-and-fast outline, no index, no table of contents. We're all authors of our own existence, constantly inventing and revising ourselves. It's up to us to choose the style of our magnum opus—Norman Mailer or Stephen King, Virginia Woolf or Judith Krantz.

> *Do not seek to follow in the*
> *footsteps of the masters.*
> *Seek what they sought.*
>
> Matsuo Basko

In my early twenties, when I was teaching high school, I was given a class of thirty-five students from ten different Spanish-speaking countries. Not one of them knew a word of English and it was my job to teach it to them. The books were late, of course, and I didn't speak a syllable of Spanish. *Chaos* reigned.

Occasionally I yelled at them in German, which would quiet them down for a few minutes. I contemplated suicide but realized that that would wipe out my entire life as opposed to just these two hours each day. And then, as I was sitting staring at a kid who was always daydreaming, I had a brainstorm: I decided to teach them English through their dreams.

Every day the kids wrote their dreams in Spanish and then translated them into English. If they didn't have a dream, they borrowed one from someone else. After reading their dreams aloud to the class, they recorded them in a huge common dream journal. God lived in these pages and these kids learned English faster than one would believe possible.

Each of us has a story and in telling this story we convert our experience into wisdom. I met a Hawaiian Kahuna with a giant heart and six kids. He told me many stories of his traditions. One that really affected me was of the Ho-O-Pono-Pono ritual. Every evening he gathers his family around him just before sunset and begins by telling them all the good things and the not-so-good things he experienced that day. Each kid does the same and it ends with the mother telling about her day. It's an opportunity to clear any unfinished business or resentments between family members. Then they sit in silence and watch the sun go down, letting all the good and the bad of their day go with it. I think often about how differently most families process their day; how many families hang onto negative events for years, leaving no space for the wisdom that flows from them.

Sometimes our stories read like mystery novels. One evening I felt absolutely called to a restaurant in Soho that we hadn't tried yet. It was a brisk winter evening and I had a craving for miso soup. The menu was a bit hard-core Japanese for my taste; nevertheless, we ordered a full-course Japanese meal. I took one bite and something hit me wrong. I couldn't continue. Since neither of us was in ecstasy about the experience and since it was a very expensive untouched meal, we had the waiter wrap it to go. We went to a restaurant further downtown and had a great meal. We left our original meal in the bag by the door in case a homeless person wandered by—all too common in this third-world country called Manhattan. When we finished our meal, the bag was still sitting there, so I picked it up in the hope we would find someone who needed food. We had walked three blocks up West Broadway when I saw a man rummaging through the garbage on the corner of Spring Street. He was bent over and I couldn't see him well at all. As he turned toward us, I asked, "Are you hungry?" He nodded yes. Before I handed him the two complete Japanese meals, I checked the bag to make sure there were chopsticks. As I lifted my head, our eyes met—he was Japanese! The first and last Japanese homeless person I have ever seen in Manhattan.

Sadly, it's in the name of God that most separation takes place. Jews are the chosen people, others are goyim (people who don't know God); Catholics go to Heaven, others languish in Purgatory or Hell; those who are born again find redemption, others don't; Muslims are believers, all others are infidels. All divisive dogmas are based on artificial hierarchies. Like I said, dogmas don't dance. In true *seeker*-consciousness, the concept of tribe and community become one. The sense of inner belonging and outer structure dissolve. There are no boundaries, no in crowds, no velvet ropes, no membership cards, no PIN numbers.

God don't make no mistakes.
That's how He got to be God.
Archie Bunker

Martha often creates art installations for my workshops that reflect the themes that we are exploring. For example, at a *Bones* gathering, on "red" day, she made an altar out of a red dress, a bowl of cherries, a fire extinguisher, a solitary red shoe, a rose, a red phone, and a stop sign. At a *Heartbeat* workshop not too long ago, she brought the hand of a mannequin and stood it in front of me and the drummers. We were only going to be in that space for one evening and then move the next morning further downtown so she wanted to do something simple. It freaked out one of my drummers, but I told him to get a grip, it was just a hand.

The next morning, to enter the new space we had to maneuver our way past a homeless couple and their two dogs who were occupying the stoop. They had been evicted the day before, and had managed to salvage only a few meager pieces of furniture and a hot plate. On the third day of the workshop, as we finished dancing sadness, someone asked if there wasn't something we could do for the family on the street below us. All of us had been touched by their presence, so we each donated some bucks and it added up to five hundred dollars. As I stood there wondering how to deliver this money, my eyes landed on the mannequin hand, our symbolic altar. It struck me to cram all the bills into the space between the fingers and send somebody down with the message, "We'd like to offer you a hand."

The dance of God goes on
without
hands and feet.
Kabir

The *seeker* lives in *chaos,* in the non-duality zone where dark and light merge in a luminous embrace. In this zone, *madonna* and *holy spirit, artist* and *lover, feminine* and *masculine,* inner and outer, all dissolve in the dance. In this frame of mind, we don't hold on, we let go. We don't think, we know. We don't do, we are. We just keep moving in the wisdom that this is our only prayer.

TO DO (or NOT TO DO)—*Seeker*

Awareness

A friend in college used to hang out in cafes in Berkeley at communal tables teaching himself how to drop his mind. His technique was simple; whatever the topic of conversation, he'd take the opposing point of view. He loved it when he had to counter his own position and argue against himself. This is a great way to practice non-attachment to beliefs, values, identity, dogmas, philosophies, and any other self-constructs. What a way to demystify yourself.

Try embracing the opposite point whenever you hear yourself taking a stand. Embrace it ardently, with the full power of your divine mind. Expand your awareness and flex those mental muscles.

Action

Think of something you feel conflicted about—whether or not to take a job, to tell someone something they don't want to hear. Start with one side of the debate. Express it through movement. Exaggerate it into a stylized dance. Now develop the other side. When both become articulated in your body, keep shifting between them in your dance. Let your attention focus on the space between them and dance this energy.

Seeker Party

You live in a community that exists within other communities. How can you offer yourself in service to one of these communities? Perhaps you can visit a home for the aged and sing or dance or read them your poetry—or get them to write their own. Maybe you could offer yourself to a hospice to do whatever needs to be done. Give one day to an organization that's making a difference. As Bob Dylan once said, "You gotta serve somebody." Who do you want to serve?

Mary Stripped of Duty

She paints
ripe light leaps through her fingertips
arching angels of deep tissue
bound by desire
claim their hue
She empties herself on to the canvas
She is the masterpiece

                              Jewel Mathieson

Chapter Seven

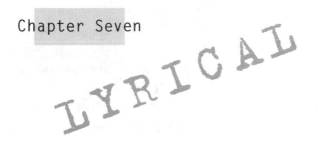

the song of a thrush or
  nightingale
spring
Balinese dancers
swinging
snowflakes
Audrey Hepburn
a field of daffodils
forget-me-nots
John Travolta in the *Michael*
  bar scene when he got all the
  women dancing with him

Calder mobiles
Matisse cutouts
frisbee
skipping rope
Tolkien
champagne
tinsel
confetti
Brahms's lullabies
jingle bells
Joan Miro—*The Constellations*

Halloween is one of my favorite holidays. I never miss the parade that twists and tumbles down Sixth Avenue through Greenwich Village like a Chinese dragon on acid. As I ran to get there on time this year, I bumped into a pair of dice wobbling down Thirteenth Street in motorcycle boots and got stuck behind a black widow spider with dangling legs and huge neon-red belly. She was walking three abreast with the "Serious Pastry" duo in business suits and lemon tart headdresses. This is Manhattan at its

most magical. There are so many colors that from the distance people look like crepe-paper streamers threading their way down the streets.

I got to the corner of Sixth and Thirteenth just in time to witness the sandwich. Two buns, a lettuce, a tomato, an onion, a beef patty, and some french fries were spread out across the avenue doing their individual dances when a whistle pierced the rabble and they all came together to make a sandwich. I cut through a crowd of screaming kids in witch costumes, tutus, and Superman capes. Oops! I stepped on Tinker Bell. A radio-station float carrying Playboy bunnies drifted by blaring Gloria Gaynor's "I Will Survive." A dozen "That Girls" with guy legs flashed smiles on cue. A drunk sailor tried to cross Sixth Avenue in the middle of a set of dominoes. He got halfway across when suddenly the dominoes tumbled down around his feet as dominoes will tend to do. He didn't have his land legs and fell down on top of them. At this point, the samba band kicked in and twin Tina Turners blew me a kiss.

The parade is the ultimate street theater, the chance to be whoever, whatever you want to be. The performers are an inspiration with their imaginative get-ups and put-downs. They work the street and those lined up on either side of it go wild with enthusiasm. Faces glow, lit up from within like pumpkins. For a few hours we are all in the same movie and it is a Cecil B. DeMille spectacular.

Lyrical is the most intricate of the five rhythms. In *flowing* we become rooted in our feminine energy; in *staccato,* in the masculine; and in *chaos,* we discover how they are integrated within us. In *lyrical* we realize we are works-in-progress. Nothing is fixed, particularly our identities. Its deeper teachings are those of self-realization, the product of detachment and fluidity.

> *Two or three things I know*
> *for sure, and one is that I*
> *would rather go naked than*
> *wear the coat the world has*
> *made for me.*
>
> Dorothy Allison

Lyrical is also the most elusive of the five rhythms. In workshops, people often say to me, "I just can't get *lyrical*." It's tough, because you can't fake it. I'm not even sure Meg Ryan could fake it. She may fake orgasms, but I bet she couldn't fake the post-coital glow.

You can't fake the aftermath of an experience if you haven't had the experience, and *lyrical* is the aftermath of *chaos*. If we don't completely let go of all the stuff we carry—the physical resistance, the emotional baggage, the mental barriers—we get stuck in *chaos*. But when we finally do divest ourselves of everything that weighs us down, we lighten up. *Lyrical* is the process of delightenment.

In our culture, people have a hard time letting go of their security blankets and letting down their defenses. Consequently, I tend to spend more time teaching *chaos* than *lyrical*. It was only recently, after twenty years of teaching, that I discovered the key to unlock *lyrical*.

Not long ago, on a warm spring evening, I led a *Waves* event in Munich with several hundred participants. We were dancing in a huge old theater hall with fabulous wooden floors and an ornately carved balcony; a high, open space with a small stage and excellent acoustics. The room was electric with anticipation before we even started. The producer had been thoughtful enough to put a small set of stairs in front of the stage so I could run up and down between the musicians and the people on the floor. I began on stage with a very jet-lagged Robert and a wild-looking Sanga in a white dashiki with a giant orange bird woven into its threads. Unlike a Manhattan gig, where everybody shows up in various shades of black, the room was a rainbow of colors.

I introduced each rhythm in my haphazard German. The dancers laughed at me but appreciated my efforts. I've become an expert at broken languages because I always try to honor the mother tongue of wherever I am teaching. It keeps me humble, in the present tense, and prevents me from wasting time waxing poetic.

Before *chaos* began I asked Jonny to demonstrate it. He went so deep so fast that his dance became an invocation and the rest of the room eagerly followed him, as if he were the Pied Piper. *Chaos* was intense; there wasn't a soul in the room holding back. Sanga's dreds were flying in all directions; Robert was in a trance—exhaustion had consumed all his resistance.

When it came time to shift into *lyrical* I didn't want to stop the energy by pausing to introduce the new rhythm, so instead I made the adjustments through the music. Robert eliminated the bass tom and established a new foot pattern using the two toms with the highest tones to lift the dancers, to lighten their steps. Sanga switched from using his hands on the djembe to using timbali sticks, but he kept the energy going with an intense, notey, highly accented song. My voice soared with them into this airy, light place. All at once, the entire tribe of dancers crossed the threshold into *lyrical*. Their bodies looked like hundreds of shimmering leaves on one huge tree. I could hear their breath and the overtones of the drums which were nestled in the high vault of the ceiling creating a symphony reminiscent of Tibetan bowls, high strings, and angelic voices.

My attention was drawn to a dancer in white who was moving as weightlessly and effortlessly as a bird. As he leapt and twirled in midair I could see the fibers of his being like light roots holding him to earth but allowing him to stretch toward heaven. His movements were whimsical, nimble, airborne—intoxicating to watch. He reminded me of a letter I had received right before I left New York from a guy named Rick in which he described what it felt like to be inside *lyrical*. "For the first time in my life it's enough just to be. I am white inner light, a simple melding of truly felt emotions, of un-baggaged spirit, of unburdened mind, of openness and freedom and fearlessness. I am a little boy riding circles in the air with outstretched arms, like a paper glider dancing the currents of the atmosphere, laughing with the breeze." And in the back corner of the room I noticed even the producer had given up all his responsibilities and was lost in a reverie of *lyrical* motion.

Lyrical is the rhythm of my spirit animal, the Raven. Ravens' aerial acrobatics fascinate us mere mortals. They're kamikazes who dive straight at the ground and at the last minute spread their wings and pull back up. Masters of wind currents, they love to fly into cliffs facing the wind and get blown and tumbled across the wild sky. Tricksters, they often fly upside down, skate across icy ponds, and hang from trees by their beaks or one foot. No wonder they've been traditionally linked to magic; their flights of fancy are playful, imaginative, and breathtaking, their iridescent wings remind us of the mystery in the dark of the void.

> *You're going to have to call*
> *us back 'cause we've gone*
> *way out today.*
>
> Zeet Peabody's
> answering machine

Lyrical is an airborne rhythm, as contrasted to *flowing* which connects us to the earth, *staccato* to fire, and *chaos* to water. To be earthy, fiery, watery, and airy is to acknowledge that we are made of all of these elements and that they inspire our outlook and actions at various times. The rhythms are the catalysts that awaken these energies within us. When our psyches take flight in the airy dance of *lyrical,* our imaginations are liberated.

We are whoever we can imagine ourselves to be. Years ago I met an American girl from the Deep South on the beach in Sitges, Spain, who fantasized about being a nanny for Princess Grace in Monaco. On a whim she mailed a letter to Her Royal Highness. A few weeks later she received an airplane ticket to Monaco for an interview. She got the job. I never forgot this story and often tell it to people who think their dreams are too wild to come true. *Lyrical* imagination is grounded in intuition which has been honed in *chaos.* Therefore we have to trust that whatever kooky schemes we come up with must have sprouted from the fertile soil of our intuitive intelligence.

It's part of growing up to know we create our own reality. We may not have control over the circumstances in our lives but we do have power over how we deal with them. Shit happens, but it's how we handle it that counts. Rather than wallow in our misfortunes, we have to take responsibility for our own lives. Victims need not apply.

In the life cycles, *lyrical* is linked with maturity. When we finally get there, we can celebrate having survived puberty and adolescence; things should be lightening up. I love asking people to recall the moment they grew up, that epiphany when they knew who they were and how they were going to play the game. "You might expect a shift like this to happen in a quiet meditation hut or out in the desert," Ya'Acov tells me. "But it happened to me at a rock concert.

"My friend's a singer in a really successful band, and I guess part of me has always envied his stardom. I was at one of his gigs surrounded by thousands of screaming teenagers. The sound was huge and the kids reached their hands out toward my friend straining to feel a wisp of his breath or a current of his movement.

"I watched and listened for a while, then I closed my eyes and put my hands over my ears. The beat rocked my body, the light show invaded my eyelids. All of a sudden, I realized that I'd spent most of my life in a fantasy, imagining myself up there on stage, feeling those hands stretched toward me, needing me. I felt something turn off inside me, some old tape. And in a wash of relief, I realized I like my life. I love my work, my family, my friends. Like a snake shedding its skin, I let go of the strain of wanting to be a star. I laughed, opened my eyes, saw my friend the rock star, and smiled at him."

For Robert, maturity struck when he was handling a mercy killing case. A twenty-six-year-old man who had been paralyzed from the neck down in a motorcycle accident had begged his twenty-three-year-old brother to kill him. He did it with a sawed-off shotgun. "When I first got the case I felt this kid's envy. He was a Polish immigrant and I had the American dream: money, success, house, kids, prestige. Meanwhile, I envied him—I couldn't imagine loving anybody enough to do what he did, to say, 'I'll go to jail for life if this is what my brother needs from me.' I looked at my life and realized I didn't have a single relationship that came close to being as deep as the one that compelled my client to commit this act of love.

"Within three months of the verdict in that trial I had terminated every relationship I had that was not supportive and essential. That's when I grew up and began to take charge of my life, identifying what was lacking in it and consciously working to fill my heart and soul rather than my mind and wallet."

Like all of the other rhythms, *lyrical* has its shadow side as well. When it's not grounded, we run the danger of getting so caught up in a fantasy or a daydream or a need to escape that we disconnect from our bodies, our hearts, and our minds and float around ourselves like a weird cloud. Several years ago I was walking down Fifth Avenue in a distracted, spaced-out mood, not paying attention to where I was going. I vaguely heard a man mutter, "This'll get you out of my way," as I felt a solid punch in my solar plexus. Suddenly I was flying through the air and landed in the gutter with a crash. My sweet Robert helped me up amidst a small circle of concerned faces. As I stood there in a state of shock, my right arm dangling like a broken wing, I watched the stranger swagger up the street as if nothing had happened. (Safety note: Beware of men wearing nothing but a t-shirt in freezing weather.) Robert said, "I'm taking you to the hospital." I looked at him as if he were crazy and replied, "No, honey, let's go have a latte and discuss it." Needless to say, Robert prevailed and I spent the night in the emergency room praying I wouldn't get an intern on the end of a thirty-six-hour shift. Being distracted and spaced out can be dangerous to your health.

TO DO (or NOT TO DO)—*Lyrical*

Lighten up. Stay in the beat of *chaos*, free and wild and rooted but lighter. Drop the effort, let go of letting go. Dance on your toes, whirling, twirling, skipping, barely touching the ground. Let yourself skip around the room, touching the air, the floor and everything else lightly. Let yourself feel whatever you feel; just hold it lightly. This is the time to feel your weightlessness, like when you bob in the water barely touching the bottom. Let the weight of the past and future drift away. Trance out but tune in. Experience the bearable lightness of your being. Focus your eyes on your fingertips and enjoy the ride.

Suggested music:

SONG	ALBUM	COMMENT
"Eternal Dance"	Totem	slow
"Ghost Dancer"	Trance	medium
"Spirit"	Waves	fast

Shapeshifter

> "I can't explain
> myself, I'm afraid, sir," said
> Alice, "because I'm not
> myself, you see."
>
> Lewis Carroll

When *lyrical* is grounded, when body, heart, and mind are working as a unit, we're not spaced out; we're perfectly tuned in. We can change channels faster than any remote control. We have the improvisational abilities of a jazz musician. The other day, for example, I sat in utter amazement in an actress friend's kitchen watching her juggle four lines on two separate phones, each with call waiting.

It all began with her mother—as things often do. She was interrupted by a call from the phone company just as the other phone rang. On that line, she talked for a moment with her best friend Buffy, who was stranded in Mexico, only to be interrupted by her agent with news of an audition. I don't know how she kept track of who was on which line, but I watched her change characters, voices, tones—everything but her costume—with the click of a button. It was an Oscar-worthy performance.

In *lyrical*, we realize that we have the freedom to keep shifting energies so as never to get stuck in any one possibility and to know that all possibilities are available to us at all times. Indeed, *lyrical* is the rhythm of the soul and the soul is a shapeshifter by nature, heir to an ancient shamanic tradition.

Legend has it that some shapeshifters could actually change their physical identities. They could make themselves invisible or transform themselves into animals. As the shaman made himself look and move like an animal by donning a costume and assuming the animal's bodily movements, something quite magical often occurred. The shaman would invoke the spirit of that animal, experience himself as that animal, and communicate insights from that animal. He would capture the creature's spiritual essence, and in doing so that essence would come to life in the hearts and minds and souls of anyone who was witness to his rite.

In modern times, the term "shapeshifting" has been all but lost. More often than not we inhabit the shadow side of the shapeshifter either trying to be invisible or trying to be somebody else. This happens when, instead of having faith in the fluidity of our own persona, we try to fix ourselves in an idea of who we are. And when we can't come up with a good idea, we imitate somebody else's. The trick is to identify with the shifting, not the shape, the process, not the product.

Shapeshifting can be a very useful concept as we explore how we can transform our lives. We have within us the capacity to change our identities by giving shape to energies trapped within us. In my dance I discovered that if I gave physical expression to a particular fear—fear of losing my lover, fear for my child's safety, fear of judgment—the fear lost its hold on me.

Shapeshifting is the key to my form of ritual theater. It's a way to dramatize the archetypal characters that dominate our lives and bring them into conscious awareness. It's as if the psyche were an anarchic theater company, composed of hams, heavies, and prima donnas with an occasional prodigy. Generally, there is no director outside of Captain Control, Herr Uber-Ego, who unfortunately has only a thimbleful of talent.

In the late sixties I signed up for a psycho-drama workshop at Esalen run by a Chinese dwarf in cowboy boots, a Subud master. I was so excited to take a theater workshop, it took several hours for the reality to wipe out my expectations. He stood before us, this tiny man with a booming voice, and announced that no one would be allowed to leave the room for any reason for the next five days. To emphasize his point, he had four assistants, each standing by a door, with a "don't even think about it" look plastered on their faces. Later we discovered they were all Aikido black belts.

The Chinese dwarf worked on each member of the group, one at a time, for hours at a stretch. He got to me on the third evening in the middle of the night. He directed five huge men from the group to hold me down. At first I fought them like a caged animal, but soon I realized it was hopeless so I gave in. But I didn't give up. I withdrew my energy and went limp. With nothing to fight against, the men relaxed, and while they were smirking and tripping on their hero dreams I slipped into the body of a snake and slithered out of their grasp. In this moment I discovered the difference between strength and power.

It wasn't over. The group formed a circle and cowboy man threw me in the center and told me to get out. I had no allies—after three days of no sleep, no food, no coffee, no smokes, no toothbrush, no friends, no change of clothes, no memories of the world as we knew it, we were like the boys in *Lord of the Flies*.

A lady did try to help me but I threw her out, not being in the mood for a mother. The other group members' faces were cold, calculating my every move. It became clear to me that there was nothing I could physically do to get out. With this realization came a strange sense of freedom; I fell to the bottom of myself and landed in my sense of humor. I started laughing hysterically, shifted totally into clown mode, and began doing somersaults, cartwheels—basically acting like a fool, but one with eyes in the back of her head. I charmed my captors into relaxing, watched their hands loosen, and spotted the weak link in the chain. I rolled out between his legs.

In the end I learned that my power was not in my physical strength but in my vulnerability. Each time I surrendered wholly to it I became empowered. I kissed the Subud master's feet for this gift and for introducing me to the shapeshifter within me.

Sometimes we need to shift in order to survive, other times the shifts take us into totally new dimensions. I remember one week in Big Sur when by day I taught a workshop and by night I crossed the Esalen property, walked through the garden with the stone scarecrow, past the round house and the waterfall house, over the bridge to the big house, and entered an alternate world, the world of Don Jose Matsuwa, a Huichol shaman.

It was an honor for me to be invited to participate in this ceremony with him. As I approached the room where the ritual was taking place, I saw him for the first time. He was far away in a mysterious song, a prayer arrow gently waving in his hand. Don Jose was over a hundred years old and looked like Neptune might after a millenium in the sea. He wore a woven band around his forehead, topped by a colorful hat. A diminutive man, his spirit filled the house, lifted the roof, and called the sky down to dance. He was sitting in front of a fire, a huge red yarn drawing depicting the shaman's journey over his head. In the center of the drawing was a peyote button, the Huichol's holy sacrament which gives them vision and heart.

We danced in a circle to the heartbeat of the drum, to the sound of the rattles, to the song of the shaman. We danced in the spirit of the deer. We danced all night every night for five nights. We danced till our feet grew wings and we became a tribe of nomads from the four corners of the world.

I danced into another dimension, a place beyond the borders of my physical self. As I moved I felt myself transforming into a raven, taking flight in a wailing wind. In the wind I heard all the things I'd never said but wanted to. It shook me to my core and scattered my parts in all directions.

In my mind's eye, I frantically picked up the pieces and placed them one by one on the altar of the Mother. They burned in her incense, ashes to dust. I wanted forgiveness but I didn't know whom to ask. I knew whom but not how. How but not when. I knew nothing. All I could do was dance round and round the circle, flying past my suffering into a luminous world.

Trance is a tricky place, a place not many understand. It's a mindful state that only happens when you get out of your way and fall into your true self so deeply that something inside clicks and you are simultaneously being and witnessing yourself. It's a myth that trance is a spell that somebody else puts you under. Trance is hypnotic but it's not hypnosis. Nobody can put you in a trance but God, and God makes you beg for it. It takes a lot of preparation to let go of being the mover and allow yourself to be moved. In a million unspoken ways, you are tested.

In trance, we move into the bigger picture. And from this vantage point we can see into the dark of our own hearts and let go of all the things that haunt us, relinquish them, turn them over to the Great Spirit. Sometimes I am moved by the spirit of raven, sometimes I am moved by the spirit of river or *madonna* or the wind. Sometimes I am moved by the spirit of fear or fury. If I let go it takes me past my ordinary self into my luminous self. Any energy fully embodied can be a gateway.

Trance is a tribal vibe; it seldom happens alone. Thank God for Paris and dingy clubs on the Left Bank, because this is where I found it for the first time outside my own dance. I observed it during a Haitian voodoo ritual in a smoky club where the priestess did all she could to dissuade us from staying. Not only were we sitting on the most uncomfortable wooden chairs ever made, but, beginning at midnight, she spent three hours drawing symbols in salt on the floor. After most of her audience had faded into the night, she began her ceremony. I was mesmerized by her intense presence, laser eyes, white robes with gold sequins, and birdlike hands, one holding a whiskey bottle and the other flickering signals in the candlelight.

As the drums began their mesmerizing beat, she slowly intoned her chants. One at a time, six young women entered and began to dance, kicking up the salt symbols and casting them to the winds. Every once in a while the priestess would take a long swig from her bottle and spit it at a dancer. As the intensity of the dancing and the drumming continued to build, ocassionally a dancer would be swept away by the hypnotic polyrhythms, her body rocking and twisting, her arms arcing in the air like a violent prayer. An hour or so after they began dancing one of the girls came barrelling straight toward me. At first I was freaked out, as she was quite heavy and I had nowhere to go to get out of her way. I put up my hand to protect myself, but at the moment of contact a strange thing occurred. I pushed her back into the circle with my index finger—she was weightless. In trance states we release all weight to the wind—mental, emotional, and physical—and surrender to the lightness of our being. In this translucent state of being we are born again.

Ten years ago, I led a workshop focusing on the marriage of art and healing at the Westerbecke Ranch in the northern California wine country. All of the participants were artists or healers. I assigned each one to make a presentation on the five rhythms through his or her particular medium. Some of the projects were visual, others were a combination of visual and performance art, still others presented the five rhythms in a teaching context. One young lady painted images of the rhythms on silk panels and turned them into lovely dance skirts, one of which I've been wearing ever since. My then-eighteen-year-old son Jonathan had said that for his project he wanted to dance his three spirit animals. He was scheduled to go last on the very last day.

I was taking a nap in my trailer trying to escape the summer heat and ubiquitous bees when Jonny came barrelling through the door filled with an electric excitement. That morning he had sat on my bed with me like a shy *madonna* in despair, as his third spirit animal still hadn't revealed itself. A friend had suggested one to him, but it didn't fit. "I can't feel it, Mom." "Go off alone and pray for the third one. It is most likely the one closest to who you are, which is why you are having such difficulty seeing it." Now he was back, bursting to tell me what he had seen.

"I walked in the foothills, through the woods, opening myself up to the universe, collecting stones, shells, bones, and feathers. Then I went back to my room and decided to meditate. From the depths of my soul I wanted my spirit animal to reveal itself to me. I sat in a full lotus, rocking and chanting until I felt this urge to call out to the Great Spirit, 'What is my spirit animal?' I reached to my right for my Medicine Cards, spread them out, and let my hand pass over them. I picked Wolf. As I stared at the card I felt euphoric. This was something I had known but couldn't trust."

Now he had his triangle of totem animals: the dolphin, the eagle, and the wolf. Traditionally, wolf is the pathfinder, the innovator, the teacher. I wasn't at all surprised that he had received his calling to the teaching path, that he would spend his life using his power to empower others. The next day we all witnessed his gift as he led the group in the most amazing movement session. He began with a very personal and poetic invocation to the four directions. He stood in the center of the circle, his long blond hair woven with feathers and twigs, his face and body painted with symbols, his soul surrendered to his mission. His arms seemed to disappear in his skin as he became a dolphin, dancing playfully around the circle which had become his ocean. Then he shifted into a majestic eagle with an enormous wingspan and our circle became his sky, his flight our prayer. Then another shift into a silver wolf. With each shift, his body transformed completely. Each dance was a prayer, a vision. He ended by gathering all of us us into his dance and leading us into trance. When it was over, I was totally dumbstruck. I had just passed the baton. A new generation of the teaching had been born.

Knowing our spirit animals is very important to our self-discovery. They link us to the animal kingdom and allow us to receive its wisdom. Each of us has a unique connection to the animal, vegetable, and mineral kingdoms of this world and these relationships are soul food. I often suggest that those who teach this work look to their spirit animals for clues as to their style of teaching. An eagle teaches very differently from a turtle or a raven or an owl. To embrace this part of yourself is to embrace a core aspect of your soul. My friend Heather is an owl and a magical storyteller. Her power turns on at night. And many a night

I've succumbed to her rhythm and found myself begging the sun to move more slowly.

While *flowing* taught us how to be part of a tribe, *staccato* taught us how to be part of a community, and *chaos* taught us how to direct the energy of those alliances into service, *lyrical* shows us our place in the universe as a whole. In *lyrical,* we seek truth about both ourselves and our mission here on this planet. No one can do this research for us, it is so highly individualized. Again and again we must reach into the unknown, mysterious part of ourself, eliminating all resistance to the creative process of self-discovery and developing the discipline to be a free spirit. To do this, we have to be willing to give up all attachment to specific identities based on gender, class, profession, sexual preference, nationality, and religion and explore ourselves as fluid fields of energy. To do this we have to drop all expectations we may be dragging with us from other times, places, and people. We have to strip ourselves bare until we unveil our naked soul.

Being in *lyrical* is like being in a zeppelin filled with a gas that is lighter than air. Our bodies, filled with soul, take flight. Up, up, and away, we move beyond the boundaries of our individual personality, we ascend above the social structures of everyday existence and witness our own unfolding.

When we're witnessing ourselves from this *lyrical* perspective, we can clearly see the landscape of the self. Archetypes are markers defining different zones of awareness and action through which we can shift. However, we must resist the temptation to become locked into them and think of them as permanent identity. Clinging to an identity is potentially lethal and we end up feeding the persona and starving the person underneath it. Take SuperMom, for example. She does her gig without X-ray vision or even a cape, juggling kids, parents, husband, job, dogs, cats, gerbils, babysitters, cleaners, Safeways. If she gets stuck in this archetype she'll collapse. She needs a hit of *madonna* meditation or a wild *son* shopping spree to balance things out.

When my friend Clare left one lover for another, she felt very guilty and kept focusing on her ex's negative traits to make herself feel better.

Only she didn't feel better. "Focus on his soul. Honor the power of his that attracted you in the first place," I suggested. "And, knowing he'll always be part of you, let him go." So she contemplated her boyfriend's archetypes: "I first loved him because under his casual charm and careful style there's a shy little girl who sits in bed with me or listens so still to a blackbird sing; a *mother* who is always wanting me to eat enough and wear warm clothes on cold days; a *father* who is present and guiding, who plays silly games in the kitchen; a crazy *son* who drives very fast through red lights and, grinning, gives policemen the finger; an *artist* who hopes and laughs and lives in the moment; a *mistress* who seduces me with long-limbed grace and a smile in his eyes; and a holy-man-ghost with hands full of love he has hidden from the world, who sees patterns and light and knows things without being told, and who changes so fast sometimes it's like magic."

Davida calls me distraught. Her dad has been diagnosed with liver failure and must wait in the hospital for a transplant. "Don't focus on his body, focus on his soul," I say to her. "Right now his body is imprisoned in a hospital gown, but his soul is constantly shapeshifting." A few days later she sends me a fax: "I took your advice. I see the *madonna* in my father when he adds a scoop of vanilla ice cream to a glass of root beer, giggling as it fizzes over the glass. His smile delights. I see the wild *son* in him as he sneaks up to the desk at the hospital and tries to put his file on top in order to be next in line. His *mistress* appears when he flirts with the nurses. I realize that these archetypes have always been present in him—I just never noticed. I used to see his *mistress* when he checked out all the women's butts at my birthday party. The wild *son* in him once took me to school and drove all the way up the steps to drop me off. The *father* in him always talks politics, letting me know the workings of the world, while the *holy spirit* in him recites *King Lear* and *Hamlet* to me."

We can view ourselves through this prism, as well, and seek out the distinct ways we inhabit the different archetypal energies. One trick is to check your closet. Our wardrobe indicates how we express these energies in the world. The part of you that shops is not necessarily the same part of you that gets dressed every day. Lots of my lady friends buy *mistress* clothes and then schlepp around in the same outfit for weeks, usually a *mother* baggy thing they can hide in. I've seen the opposite too. I was admiring my young friend Cherie's vinyl pants the other day. "Mercy, little sister, those pants are hot!"

"Aren't they cool?" she responds. "My *mistress* is vinyl. I have g-string vinyl underwear, these vinyl pants, a vinyl jacket—sometimes I think my brain is vinyl! But I'm not stuck there. You should check out my *father* power suits, they're commando outfits that zip up and have collars. And my *son* is into cut-offs and flannel shirts, anything ripped. Funny, I figured out the other day that my *holy spirit* energy is into jeans and backpacks, not halos and robes."

These energies also reside in places which become their power spots. My *mother* energy loves my big blue bathtub, my birth mother's *mother* is at the kitchen table, my son's *mother* is on a massage table, and my husband's *mother* hangs out on the beach.

Once we find out where they're hiding and what they're wearing, it's time to party, to celebrate all the facets of who we are. Turn up the music and let them all dance.

TO DO (or NOT TO DO)— *The Shapeshifter*

Awareness

Which archetype decorated your living space? *Madonnas* have wall-to-wall altars. *Mothers* have comfortable chairs with ottomans to put their feet up. *Fathers* have functional furniture that's not necessarily comfortable. Wild *son* might live in a tent or a tree house or on the edge of a cliff overlooking the wild surf. *Mistress* is lace, satin sheets, soft lights, velvet couches, fur throws. *Holy spirit* lives in a monk cell with a futon on the floor, frame not included, one reading lamp, a pile of books, and a hot plate.

Who bought your car? The difference between a *father* car and a *son* car can be dramatic. Who takes taxicabs, prefers the bus, or likes to walk?

What part of you relates to nature and what part of nature do you relate to? Do you need wide open spaces and vistas, pounding surf, or heavily wooded forests? Deserts or mountains? Fields where things grow or empty lots you can build on? My *madonna* draws me to nature, whereas my surf-baby Jonny's wild *son* draws him. Kathy's *holy spirit* defines her relationship to nature. Different environments call upon different parts of us. Some of us are drawn to the stars, others to archeological digs, some to study animal behavior, while others are fascinated by human nature.

Action

Fast-forward through on your life, beginning with your infancy. Do your baby dance—use the floor. When ready, break into your toddler dance, then let yourself wobble into childhood, reviving all those child games and playing with your imaginary friends. Feel the g-force of puberty propel you to move into goofy, giddy, hormone-charged dances. Think high school—need I say more? Keep going, let yourself waltz into maturity and do your responsible, get-it-together, take-charge dance until you're bone tired, then drop into the sweet surrender of your slo-mo dance.

Recycle yourself, letting go of your past, the negative shapes you harbor, the emotional baggage you carry. It's environmentally sound.

Service

Sit on your couch—if you don't have one, a pillow will do—and ask yourself the question: Where can I make a difference? Who can I offer myself to as a companion for an afternoon, or evening or whatever? Is there a bored kid, lonely elder, overwhelmed parent, or someone struggling with a disability who could use my love and support? Reach out and touch someone.

My Spirit Takes the Wind
by Surprise

These endless permutations of sand
These endless permutations of being
To be . . . To be like the child
that clasps a piece of glass and talks it into being a diamond
I'm looking . . . I'm looking for that perfect shade of purple
   to dye my eyes in
   and sweep the sky with my lashes

Jewel Mathieson

Chapter Eight

STILLNESS

Captain Picard	library
jellyfish	orchids
Butoh dancers	Thich Nhat Hahn
Buddha	rocks
empty church	sleeping cat
Arvo Part	snake
Marlon Brando	Yoda
zero	turtle
Kauai	cloister convent
Owl	Arc de Triomphe
mime	Picasso's Blue Period
pyramids of Gaza	"Sketches of Spain" by Miles
archery	Davis
desert	

T erry and I stroll over to the Coffee Shop on Union Square for a Brazilian lunch. Inside rock music blares and the wait-people are all exotic model types. We squeeze into a booth and over a veggie burger and a barbecue chicken sandwich discuss *The Wizard of Oz* as a metaphor for the spiritual journey.

As we leave the restaurant we spot two huge buses parked across the street. Filing out is a huge contingent of Tibetan Buddhist monks with shaved heads, ochre and crimson robes, and sandals. Each one claims a suitcase from the belly of the bus and walks across the square to the Zen Palate restaurant. "We don't have to go to the Himalayas anymore," Terry says. "They're coming to us."

Across from the farmer's market we notice a mime posed on a plastic milk crate with a sign hanging off it: "Donations make the still life move." The mime is a vision in silver, from his hightops up through his baggy pants and flowing tunic to every inch of his black skin. His hair is silver with three black stripes and he has on black shades.

I throw a dollar into the box to activate the coin-operated silver man. His face lights up, his red tongue slips out, and he leaps off the crate. He takes a seed from his heart, plants it in the sidewalk, watches intently while the flower emerges from the concrete, snips it, and hands it to me.

As crowds of people stop to stare, he creates an aura of utter *stillness*. The ripples and waves in his hands and the swivel of his hips unite us in fascination. His moves are precise and mechanical, yet totally fluid. Watching him I am reminded that we are ninety percent water. He stoops, looks in a small mirror, powders his silver brow, and leaps back on his crate, then he slides his hands down his ribcage to his hip bones, leans his head forward, and and reassumes his stone-still pose.

"Believe it or not I learned to meditate in this crazy city," I said, turning to Terry. When I lived in Big Sur, I had to struggle to meditate. Everything outside me was slow and still, while inside I felt all revved up. When I came to Manhattan in the early seventies, life reversed itself: outside it was loud and fast, so if I wanted *stillness* I had to take refuge in myself. Somewhere deep within me I found the quietest spot in Manhattan."

These days I love to sit in Washington Square Park and contemplate the mysteries of our existence. The rhythms, the archetypes, the cycles, the waves—all of it is in the park on any given day. I sit still and a guy flows by on Rollerblades with a silver dog on a leash. *Mistress* is the kid plugged into his Walkman singing a Snoop Doggy Dog tune at full volume. I see *madonna* in the young man sitting next to me reading a book and in the chess players intent on every move. The policeman saunters by like big daddy surveying his kingdom. Wild *son* rides a skateboard, leaping over a garbage can and astonishing the *holy spirit* Hasidim handing out red-and-white pamphlets entitled, "The Weekly Publication for Every Jewish Person."

It's all happening at once—I contemplate the brilliance of *chaos*. Meanwhile, the *artist* is everywhere. Two N.Y.U. students sit on the bench nearby and begin filming a couple across from them, while a guy strums a guitar behind me. A girl in full *seeker* mode meditates in a full lotus on the grass, and an elderly lady in a bright yellow bonnet is nodding off and not even the screaming child next to her can shake her from the *stillness* of her dream.

The first time I experienced *stillness* in my dance was after the *lyrical* trance/dance I did in the Huichol ceremony back in Big Sur. After the deer dance, I stopped and sat on the hardwood floor amidst dozens of people shaking rattles and chanting haunting, high-pitched ancient melodies. My spine was writhing and the rattles echoed in my head. I could see that my foot was bleeding, but I couldn't feel it. It seemed as if I were looking at my foot from the other side of the world; totally detached from my body, yet more deeply rooted in it than I had ever been. Each breath was like a giant wave rolling through me and crashing against the imaginary boundaries of my body.

The mystery revealed me to myself as simply a moving meditation: I had to move to find the *stillness*; I had to stop dancing to feel the dance. Eventually, I was drawn back into a circle of dancers but within me I had found a whole new range of motion. Every move was subtle, almost as if each cell of my body were a universe unto itself.

Tim, the lead singer of one of my favorite rock bands, is looking a bit like an alien angel since he shaved his head. Over dinner I asked if he was vying for membership in the wounded healer club. His trademark is wild, *chaotic* dancing, and while on tour recently, he ruptured a disc and had to wear a neck brace. "I had no idea when I titled the album *Whiplash* that strange forces would be set loose. The title for my next album is going to be *I Won the Lottery,*" he mused. To make up for not being able to dance wildly he pushed his voice and the next day woke up with a strained larynx. That night he had to perform in a neck brace with a weak voice. "I couldn't do any of my tricks. I couldn't dazzle them. All I could do was be there. Yet, the audience was more connected to me than ever. My voice had more resonance and presence—I sounded better than I ever had. I had tapped into an exquisite power in my vulnerability which was totally unexpected. For the first time I understood the difference between the power of being and the power of doing."

On the night Robert Kennedy was shot, I had been invited to a party for the grandson of Haile Selassie, then the emperor of Ethiopia. It was too late to call the party off so my Ethiopian friends decided to have the party in silence out of respect for a fallen hero. The Ethiopians carried this off with dignity and grace, moving about the room like tree people, sitting, eating, and simply being. The Americans invited to the party, however, were uncomfortable and self-conscious, giggling, twitching, and constantly going out on the balcony for cigarettes where they could whisper in defiance. It was embarrassing to see how threatened we were by silence.

Westerners seem to be afraid of *stillness* and silence. We come into our homes, take off our Walkmans or throw down our portable phones, and switch on the TV even if we have no intention of watching it. It's as if we were programmed to fill every empty space with noise and activity. We seem to be afraid that if we leave a gap something inside of us might bubble up and take us off guard. Maybe we're really afraid of the silence of the grave; death is, after all, the ultimate *stillness.*

> *Either this wallpaper goes or*
> *I do.*
> Oscar Wilde, on his deathbed

As we approach death, we move in the rhythm of *stillness.* A few weeks ago, Jonathan and I were in a taxi on our way to a workshop uptown. On Twenty-third and Sixth, the cab screeched to a halt as a frail wisp of a woman who must have been in her eighties was crossing the street. The light changed three times before she reached the opposite sidewalk. Meanwhile traffic backed up and horns blared. Jonny reached over and grabbed my hand, "See, Mom? *Stillness.*" I felt both a profound compassion for and inspired by this woman. How courageous of her to be maneuvering Manhattan and quietly going about her business in her winding-down period of life.

Kathy tells me, "In their eighties, my parents are both the same and different from the people I've always known. My father still reads voraciously, but it takes him a week to finish a book he would've polished off in a night. He still paints but now he only paints during sunny days, when the weather permits his failing eyes to see the true colors and his hands are warm enough to stay steady. He still walks the same streets he walked as a young salesman but his pace is slowed. He's been married to the same woman for sixty-four years. They still bicker constantly, but even that has taken on the feel of an old worn cashmere sweater. Up until a few years ago he insisted on carrying my suitcases from taxi to curb; now he doesn't put up such a fight. He is surrendering to this *stillness* cycle, as he must, but he's not happy about it.

"Making soup used to be easy for my mother; now it's a big deal. She is no longer able to shop and cook on the same day, needs to sit between dicing and sauteeing. When all is prepared and finally shimmering on the stove, the aroma coaxing you into believing that everything is as it was, my mother pads to the bedroom and falls into an exhausted sleep. Napping has become an essential ingredient of her afternoons.

"I feel my mother straining to do more, find her old stamina, but she is at the mercy of her body and the weather. She studies Shakespeare and short stories, reads the *Times* from cover to cover and can still answer the final *Jeopardy* question correctly. But like a leaf clinging to a branch in fall, her hold is fragile, her grip tentative."

We don't have to wait till we're eighty-seven to experience *stillness*. We contain our future within us. Any time we are ready we can access the lessons of *stillness*: wisdom, compassion, and inspiration. These are embodied by the archetype of the *alchemist*.

Not so long ago Robert received a call from a dying friend requesting that we come to the hospital. When we got there, Robert didn't recognize her and walked right by her bed—she had shrunk from a robust statuesque beauty queen to a sliver of bones. In spite of her weakness, she was in good spirits for our visit. Before we left she handed each of us an envelope with our specific assignment for her funeral: she wanted Robert and me to deliver her eulogy.

She had choreographed the entire event, including the selection of the funeral parlor. She personally visited every one in her area and picked out the homiest one. She gave instructions for each friend to do what they did best. She asked one to do her makeup and hair the night of her death and another she gave a present to give her daughter on her twenty-first birthday. To yet another she assigned the task of giving away her possessions. One friend was in charge of the party and Vivian's spirit permeated every detail, from the food to the music to the ambience. It was truly a celebration with no space for indulgence or even mourning, just the way she wanted it.

Turning this negative event of her death into a beautiful work of art that wove all those she loved into a tapestry of beauty, love, friendship, and creativity—instead of maudlin sentiment or a dead ritual that had nothing to do with her—was the work of the *alchemist* in her soul. It was as much a celebration of her life as it was an honoring of her death.

TO DO (or NOT TO DO)—*Stillness*

Slow down. Move in super-slow motion. Gather your energy inward. Sink into the emptiness. Disappear in the dance. Occasionally stop and feel your shape. Watch your breath. If your mind is chattering, do some quick moves between stops.

Let your arms float like clouds around your body as you shift your weight from one foot to the other. Settle into the stops, like a mime. Your dance looks like a series of snapshots with movement in between.

Slowly come to rest. Sit. Close your eyes. Focus your attention on the ebb and flow of your breath, the beat of your heart, the pulsing of your cells. And in this womb of stillness, in this song of silence, embrace the mystery that is you.

It's all a prayer.

Suggested music:

The album *Stillpoint* offers a variety of expressions of this rhythm, as does *Devi* by Chlöe Goodchild.

Alchemist

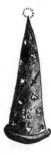

*I merely took the energy it
takes to pout and wrote some
blues.*

Duke Ellington

After my car accident in Spain, when I was in London teaching and being treated by my Tibetan Buddhist osteopath, I had another little mishap. The heel of my weathered ankle-boot got caught on the hem of my wide-legged Ghost pants and I crashed to the ground, splitting open the back of my already-concussed head.

A waif of a girl with bright red hair helped me up. She and her boyfriend, in weary leather with nails protruding through his cheeks, carried me to my hotel. Blood running down my face, I looked akin to Jesus with his crown of thorns.

It was too late to call off my evening workshop. I had just enough time for an emergency visit to an acupuncturist and then I was up on the stage again, standing before a few hundred dancing maniacs. I had two long acupuncture needles sticking out of the top of my throbbing head as I stared out at the bodies waiting for my next move. I had no moves; all I could do was sing. I poured myself into the song, turning desperately to the mournful melody—it was all that held me up. "Yanna wanna yana ho ey O yana."

Two evening events, two weeks in a row, two serious accidents—I knew somebody was trying to get through to me. I was supposed to be in London to teach workshops, not to be torn limb from limb. I couldn't help feel that the two were somehow connected—what I had to teach and what I had to learn.

> *Only two things are infinite,*
> *the universe and human*
> *stupidity, and I'm not sure*
> *about the universe.*
> *Albert Einstein*

I'd arranged for live music that night. As the recorded warmup music played, The Band of Holy Joy set up their instruments on the stage behind me: traps, tablas, violin, and synthesizer. They began to play and an assistant faded out the tape. Soon the room was filled with the eerie strains of the violin, crisscrossed by intricate tabla patterns and a synthesizer program that sounded like ten thousand monks chanting in tongues.

I scanned the room, taking in the thin doctor who studies infectious diseases, the rock star in his girlfriend's little black dress, the girl with fiery eyes whose every move is a warning to keep your distance, the construction worker with the long, lonely face, the public relations goddess whose life is parodied in a popular English sitcom, the social worker with the sunken chest who dances in black Reeboks, the philanthropist who looks like Moses and dances like Job, the poet in a knee brace, the ski instructor from Utah, the opera director flirting with him. As I watched, they all slowly dissolved into one huge sea of bodies, bending and twisting in the hypnotic beat.

Normally, I would be giving instructions and dancing too. But in my freaked-out, vulnerable state I could only sit and watch. Unable to move, I let all the waves of energy circling the room move through me. In spite of my concussion and my gash, I was more conscious and fully present than ever—almost as if I had been knocked into an altered state.

In this *God, Sex, & the Body* workshop, we were exploring the feminine and masculine rhythms, dancing the archetypes of *mother, mistress, madonna, father, son,* and *holy spirit.* The band broke into the *flowing* rhythm and I urged the room to take on the spirit of *mother.* About thirty minutes into the session, I felt bewildered—I was looking out at an army of Donna Reeds. This wasn't unusual, but for the first time I realized that there was something wrong with this picture. Without the distraction of my own dance, I was forced to notice how far away the dancers were from any sense of truth. It was scary how stuck they were in stereotypes.

As I sat there in my *stillness* contemplating the dancers, I felt the archetypal spirit of *mother* moving through the room, swirling around the bodies like a wild wind, but for the most part disembodied. Without the spirit moving within them, the dancers in the room looked disconnected from their bodies. How was I going to seduce *mother* back into our bodies? More to the point, how was I going to seduce *mother* back into my own body? A person in my condition shouldn't have been out of bed, much less teaching a workshop. But there I sat, ready to mother the entire world even as I denied myself the same caring and nurturing.

I sat there in utter despair, swirling in surreal hopelessness. The despair wasn't just in me, however; I felt it reverberating through the entire room. Clearly, there was something missing from the dance. I could feel it out there somewhere, formidable in its absence, like the phantom pain from a lost limb.

Sitting in my own state of shock and grief, unable to move my body and take refuge in the dance, I saw the desperate *mother* archetype expressed in the collective body of the room. I glimpsed her face, felt her shape, smelled her sweat, and saw how our denial of her power has kept us frozen, numb, on edge, and suspended in a never-never land, neither dark nor light.

I had a brainstorm—all the bullshit must have fallen out the crack in my head. I suggested that the dancers dive into their own darkness, into the shadows that haunted their dreams, into the devouring *mother* they were all trying so hard to repress. I signaled to the band for more intensity. A bigger, badder, harder beat.

Something shifted. Suddenly the room came alive! The energy kicked in and the whole place vibrated with the group's recognition of the shadow *mother*. They crossed an invisible portal into psychic territory, an underground place that was familar yet rarely explored, the realm of Kali, mother deity of Hindu mythology, goddess of death, destruction, and eternity. We'd peeled back the filmy veil that separated us from this other reality and and found the gateway to the dark side of the moon. And we all knew that we knew this place all too well.

Masks cracked, smiles hung lopsided, eyes turned inward, wet hair flew in all directions. Winged feet carried bodies to the other side, to the invisible side of life where all is spirit and spirit is all there is. I could see right through the dancers to the soulful self in each of them. And in each soul I saw an alchemist working his magic, bringing them to the place of wonder, awe, and mystery they were all seeking.

From the very beginning I'd always felt this workshop was a map revealing—if nothing else—how little we know of the soul. But it had divulged a new secret: when our spirit is separated from our flesh, our soul shrinks within our body, withering to a tiny, dormant seed. I thought of the seeds found in ancient Egyptian tombs, still viable, ready to burst into life after ten thousand years in the sterile void.

My fall—the injuries from the car accident and splitting open my head on the sidewalk—had grounded me in the observer position from which I was witnessing the true outcome of our collective fall from grace. How did we ever get so stuck in our ideas of what it means to be a man or a woman? What happened to the feminine spirit in each of us? I thought about Adam and Eve, the spirits of man and woman basking in the sheer bliss and mystery of life. What had we learned? What legacy did Eve pass on to all of us the day she ate the forbidden fruit?

For me, Eve's legacy—the fall from grace that she shared with Adam—is the metaphor for our collective wound. It is a legacy of dismemberment, the separation of spirit from flesh. In this state of being divided against ourselves, we became vulnerable to the onslaught of the ego.

Ego is all the voices in our heads chattering like a bunch of soap opera characters; all those divas, demons, and doyennes dripping with diamonds telling you that you aren't rich enough, smart enough, beautiful enough, talented enough, sexy enough—or that you're more of the above than anyone else, only the world hasn't discovered it yet. These voices drown out the song of the soul, the part of us that has no identity to protect or viewpoint to project.

What I learned in this workshop was that there is no way out but through. To get in touch with pure archetypal energies we have to dance their shadow side as well as their light. We have to put on our Stetsons and become J. R. Ewing, put on our stilettos and become Alexis Carrington. The only way to deflate our ego characters is to inflate them, then burst their bubbles. Instead of avoiding them or letting them intimidate us, we have to inhabit our ego characters and ham them up. Only then will we realize how ridiculous they are and how pathetic we are in our subservience to their demands.

Just as an alchemist spins dross into gold, by dancing the dark we transform it to light. Negative energy and suffering become mere grist for the mill. In the dance, we discover parts of us we've cast in the shadows and by bringing them into the light we diffuse their power over us. In the shadows *mother* is smothering and devouring. *Mistress* is numb, pissed off, and depressed. *Madonna* is manipulative and obsessive. *Father* is overbearing and rigid. *Son* is destructive, aimless, and uncommunicative. *Holy Spirit* is judgmental and dogmatic. In the shadows the *artist* is an imitator and a predator who relies on the creativity of others. The *lover* is abusive and frigid. And the *seeker,* of course, founds a commune and becomes a guru.

Geordie is a very together woman, an accomplished dancer, terrific mother, fabulous masseuse—someone who has spent her whole life in tune with the rhythms of her body. She came to a recent *Bones* workshop ready to dive into her shadow. After a very intense movement session, I asked people to sit in *stillness* with a partner and tell them, "What it is that you want to let go of?" Geordie said, "This incredible blood-curdling, earsplitting scream I feel trapped inside my chest like a stone in my heart."

In the next part of the workshop I assigned them to write on the theme of "bones." Geordie produced this poem:

CRONE

Burns burns she burns in my bones
She is taking me taking me home

She cackles and hisses and spits and curses
She stirs her cauldron with feelings and kisses
She dances the stone dance inside of my heart
She is Kali and Pele and Crone

Crone crowning the Queen in all women
You'll find her by full moon, in firelight and screaming
She wants to be speaking she wants to be screaming
Her wild witch-like cackle, her howl at the moon

Dark Queen of the night in my blood and my bones
And I honor her dance through my veins
Take me oh take me I'm yours lady death

Though I tremble and quake at your door
Here is no turning back for this lady in black
For this wonderful temptress who burns

Burns burns she burns in my bones
She is taking me home,
BURNS BURNS SHE BURNS IN MY BONES
SHE IS TAKING ME TAKING ME HOME

After the writing exercise we broke up into small ritual theater groups. Geordie's group chose to choreograph her poem. She performed this poem with burning intensity, her voice strong and clear. A chorus joined in the last lines, bursting into a maniacal hag cackle which shattered the room. I knew this was the scream that had been trapped inside her chest. Her *alchemist* was at work, first dancing until she felt her stone heart, then articulating it through her poem, releasing it through her performance, and finally transmuting the screaming witch into a powerful crone.

A month later, Geordie called me from California. "You're never going to believe this, Gabrielle, but I swear as the body is my bible that it's true. For three weeks after the workshop, I experienced the most bizarre phenomenon. These teeny tiny grains of stuff—it felt like sand to me—kept secreting out of my skin, especially where I sweat, down my back, my chest, my belly. I went to the doctor in a panic and he said he'd never seen anything like it before but I seemed perfectly healthy to him and not to worry. Finally, I figured out what it was. It was that stone heart inside me all ground up and being pushed out of my body."

The *alchemist* breaks the tape loop of our obsessive thinking. Before Eva discovered her preference for women, she knew there was something not happening in the state of Denmark. After a particularly intense workshop she spent two weeks hiding out in the dance studio next to her house, cut off from her family and friends. "My mind spun the web of all that was wrong. I was trapped in an isolated area, married to a dear friend, not a lover, and barely in touch with my numb and aging body. My mind was obsessively turning, not as a Dervish to God, but as Tragedy Queen to Despair. Chain-smoking in darkness, I wrote haiku to the God I couldn't feel.

Please fill the hole
I can't stand the emptiness
Another minute.

"Then I got up and started dancing—I didn't even bother with music. Instead of being afraid of the empty hole I dove right into it. I thought to myself, Alice did it—why can't I? I danced and I danced until the hole became holy, until the emptiness became sacred space."

Instead of running from our fears, we must have the courage to stop and get to know them. Only then can we overcome them; only then will those fears that have been ingrained in us and become part of our egos lose their grip. The other day in a restaurant, my waitress was so angry she was trembling. But she managed a terse little smile and asked me what I wanted. What I really wanted was to stop everything, put on some angry music like Nine Inch Nails, crank up the volume to the max, and urge her to dump all her anger into a dance. Instead I ordered a salad and a cup of Earl Grey Tea.

It was sad that this young woman was so identified with one part of herself that it had swallowed the rest of her up into a bad attitude. I didn't know her and she didn't know me, but I knew her anger, I knew her situation, and I knew she wasn't fooling anyone with her tight little smile. Her anger, no matter how nice she tried to be, guided her voice and shaped her body and mind, guaranteeing her a bad day.

Before we put ourselves back together we have to allow ourselves to all apart. But we don't have a clue how to do that, and we're not sure who we'd be or how we'd live our lives if we did. These are the kinds of things we're really longing to know. We're longing to be bigger than all the seemingly disparate parts of ourselves—the angry person, the smiling one, the one who's resentful, and the one who truly wants to be helpful, responsive, and loving. We're longing to overwhelm our ego, with all its pathetic complaints, comparisons, and competitions.

> *I thank God for*
> *all the things I*
> *don't have.*
> St. Teresa of Avila

So how do we shrink all those petty tyrants down to size if we don't have a little bottle handy labeled "Drink Me"? This is where awareness and attention become our allies. We can be aware of our competitive thoughts or greedy covetings, but not give them any attention. In other words, don't feed the monster, starve it. When you're aware that you're feeling competitive, this awareness gives you a choice; you can pay attention and give your energy to that feeling or shift your focus into creative action. Me? I dance.

Envy, boredom, and all of the other districts of egoland are just energy fields that we must pass through. These attitudes aren't personal unless and until you attach yourself to them; it's not the energy but the attachment to the energy that is deadly. Movement is the antidote to attachment.

It's not the conscious awareness of shadow energies that is your enemy, as painful as it may be at first, but the unconscious acting out of them. Ignorance is not bliss in my book.

We have to take off our rose-colored glasses; life is not a sitcom. Then again, it's not a funeral. We've all been wounded, even if you haven't been invited to tell us about it on daytime TV. It's time to get over ourselves, hang up our crosses, and get on with it. I'm sick of hearing us define ourselves only in terms of our wounds, forgetting that we also contain the power to heal ourselves.

The *alchemist* takes our pain and turns it into compassion for ourselves and for each other. This is the part of us that contains our power to overcome even the most horrendous abuse. I'm always astonished when I hear interviews with Holocaust survivors who are upbeat, accomplished, and fully engaged with life rather than wallowing in the victim role. They draw on the *alchemist* within them.

Astronomers tell us that most of the universe is made up of invisible missing mass known as dark matter. Some of them see light coming out of this dark matter. I do. And in the stillpoint of this light I see the *alchemist* spinning fear into love and pain into prayer.

TO DO (or NOT TO DO)— *The Alchemist*

Awareness

You are an *alchemist* capable of turning your pain into art, transforming negativity into creativity, anger into compassion. Face it—you need garbage to make compost.

It takes commitment to traverse mountains of bullshit in the dark; there's no way out but through. You'll also need a sense of humor, trust me.

What is the nature of your hidden reality? What do you sweep under the rug, shove in the closet, or let simmer on the back burner? What's behind your inertia, held in your rigidity, mashed in your confusion? What causes you to space out or black out? What emotional baggage are you carrying? Has your fear turned to paranoia, your anger to blame, your sorrow to depression? Do you diminish your joy? Are you a thousand-watt bulb amped down to a hundred? What shadow characters star in your soap opera? To whom have you given your power? Who do you want power over?

Without sinners, who would need saints?

Action

Even the rhythms have their shadow sides. Without music, do your inertia dance—let it carry you into your *flowing* vibe. Do your rigid, tense, uptight *staccato* dance until you break through to your pulse, your passion, your playfulness. Dance your confusion, your scattered brain, your panic until it releases you into *chaos*. Do your spaced-out, whacked-out, ditzy dance until you land in *lyrical*. Investigate catatonia, its shapes, its numbness, its dead weight—do your dead-can't-dance number until it empties you into *stillness*.

Repeat at least a thousand times!

The Shadow Party

Have a "dark side of the moon" party. Only the shadow knows how to dress for this occasion. Invite everyone to be downright dark. For example, dress up as their fearsome or fearful showoff or shy-away, pleaser or pouter, villian or victim character. Be creative. Break out. Camp it up. This is a party to lure the shadow into the light.

Creative suggestions: Do the whole party in candlelight; take black-and-white photos; hang a sheet from the ceiling, backlight it and have a shadow-people show. Have a game of shadow charades where people guess your character's favorite phrase. Have a Lenny Bruce Award for the darkest humor or an Anne Rice Award for the character least able to deal with the light.

To the Lies That Become Us

This body is for asking
This body is for asking those questions
   that do not live in the mind
These questions have a life of their own
   or death

Burial grounds in the heart my friend
A shovel and a map
Dig anywhere
The treasure is everywhere

This body is the answer
This body is for emptying
This body is for emptying into ether
   for opening into psyche-scapes only tip-toed around
This body is for seducing
This body is for seducing self and god-given truths back into
   matter
This body is to hold
This body is to hold, to house the sacred city of the soul

Light up. Light up these cells
Sadness has come to open all the windows
   To open all the doors

These things happen
These things happen when you make your bones your home
When each footprint becomes an altar left
   for the next dancer's self-sacrifice

                                        Jewel Mathieson

Chapter Nine

WAVES

I love waves; I wish I had some in my hair. My daddy did, but I guess I didn't dive into that end of the gene pool. Virginia Woolf wrote my favorite book, *The Waves,* and I have a son who surfs them. I danced a thousand dances to Patti Smith's song "Wave" and I've waved a thousand good-byes. I've seen waves come and take my house, flood the same bedroom where they accompanied countless nights of lovemaking. I have ridden the waves of labor, of sorrow, and of bliss.

I look at the rhythms as a wave, a continuous flow of energy, each one containing the others. The Wave of the five rhythms is my path, my practice, and my perspective.

The Wave of the rhythms is the key to the entire creative process, whether you are having a baby, choreographing a dance, designing a building, directing a play, or having an orgasm. For example, I'll start gathering ideas for an album, mulling over them, rolling them around, allowing them to percolate (*flowing*). If I honor this process the ideas will begin to form themselves into songs (*staccato*). I enter the studio confident that it will all fall apart, and it almost always does (*chaos*). If I allow the forces of plan and process, form and substance, Robert and Gabrielle to complete their dance, the album will emerge in a new light with a direction of its own (*lyrical*). The big ah-ha at the end of the tunnel is to have an album in my hand, the sweet *stillness* of completion.

As a practice I know that however hard something is I can let it go in my dance and my dance will support me. It keeps me loose and flexible. It liberates me from any fixed notions of how I think things should be. It keeps me fascinated, on my toes, open to change, alert, and intuitive.

The five rhythms are a map to everywhere you want to go, on all planes of consciousness—inner and outer, forward and back, physical, emotional, and intellectual. They are markers on the way back to a real self, a vulnerable, wild, passionate, instinctive self. A self worth dying a thousand ego-deaths for, to embody, embrace, and emancipate your soul.

Vinnie writes to me: "Funny thing happening to me with the rhythms; seems as if they are becoming a vehicle by which I know myself. I don't even think of them anymore as something I do; rather, they are what I am becoming."

In *flowing* you discover yourself. In *staccato* you define yourself. *Chaos* helps you dissolve yourself, so you don't end up fixed and rigid in the self you discovered and defined. *Lyrical* inspires you to devote yourself to digging deep into the unique expression of your energy. And *stillness* allows you to disappear in the big energy that holds us all so you can start the whole process over again.

To help you see how integral these rhythms are to everyday life, I wanted to leave you with writings I've gathered from my friends and students, as well as some of my own, each describing a wave in their life journey. Some are poetic, some linear, some discursive; all are meant to encourage you to open yourself up to seeing life from this perspective.

Subway Wave—*Gabrielle*

On a recent Sunday morning, after shopping at J & R for computer supplies, I got on the N train at City Hall. There were just a few people in the car, singles and couples coming into town from Brooklyn. The vibe was clearly laid back. I fell into my subway trance, listening to the sound of the wheels and feeling the slow, *flowing* rocking of the train.

Several groups of Chinese folk got on at Canal Street, in Chinatown, and the entire feel of the car changed to *staccato* as they animatedly conversed in short phrases at a high decibel level. Kids were running and jumping up and down the aisle. I played hide and seek with one who would hide behind her mom's skirt.

At Prince Street, a bunch of teenage girls got on, chattering, giggling, teasing, dissing, screaming over the jungle music playing on their boom box. They drowned out the poor Chinese, who stared at them in amazement. As we pulled into Eighth Street the teenyboppers realized they were going uptown when they wanted to be going downtown and suddenly the *chaos* peaked with girls pushing, shoving, pulling, shrieking as they got off with the bewildered Chinese families.

As the train pulled away, a violin player in khakis, white sneakers, a silver clipped David Niven mustache, and a dirty white golf cap entered from the next car and serenaded me and the remaining couple from Brooklyn with a *lyrical,* semi-classical song. Right before the next stop he walked his cup up and down. As I put my dollar in, I noticed he had a twinkle in his eye.

At Union Square I exited to an empty platform. The train pulled away leaving me in a stone-still silence and *stillness.*

Hiking Wave—*Eliezer Sobel* (writer)

Climbing Big Sur mountain after dancing the five rhythms all week, I see them play out perfectly in the movement of my legs on the ground. The ascent is slow and steady, strong and *flowing,* pushing through inertia with increased breath and feeling the contact between my feet and the earth. Later, coming down, gravity and I become more energized and I begin walking faster and with a sort of "left, right, left, right" regularity, exhaling with each step, spontaneously hiking in *staccato.* And then, it's getting dark, and at some place in the trail I suddenly find myself leaping forward in a sort of free-for-all downhill slalom run, crashing through branches, falling on my backside and sliding down a mossy ravine. I'm running down a mountain in *chaos* at night, and yet I feel utterly safe, because I've learned to dance inside that rhythm so that the very path I'm walking on feels like my dance partner. On level ground, at the bottom, I feel the light and *lyrical* joy of arriving, of having made it. I run and skip toward the fresh Big Sur mountain stream, where I finally collapse in the *stillness* of drinking water like a deer in the forest.

Relationship Wave—*Gabrielle & Robert*

Courtship
     Commitment
          Collison
               Communion
                    Confluence

Memorial Wave—*Chris Donovan* (nurse)

Early Saturday morning I drive in the steady flow of city traffic to the cemetery. My friend has invited me to the one-year memorial service for her stillborn son. Once inside the iron gates, I slowly circle around the thin ribbon of road. I pass statues and gravestones shaded by ancient evergreens as I find my way to the chapel enclosed in a massive mausoleum.

Inside it is stone quiet, and I can hear the pulsing beat of my heart. As I walk the straight and narrow marble hallways, the clicking of my heels becomes a rhythm of life echoing in the profound stillness of death. I am struck by my own mortality. Behind flickering votives, the priest says that the first and last second of life belong to God. The grandfather hands me a holy card. The father hands me a rose.

After the service, the parents lead everyone outside to walk to the children's burial area and their baby's grave. As we arrive, the grandmother observes that there are many new grave sites since last year. She softly speaks of wandering in cemeteries with her daughter, comforting themselves and other mothers they found who had lost loved ones. I listen, surrounded by many tiny graves, each one uniquely decorated. I am drawn to one haphazardly covered with faded storybooks, weathered stuffed animals, toys, and a gold angel. It is as if the child had emptied out his toybox and then disappeared. These images dissolve my composure and I begin to sob, my tears falling on the earth holding the children.

The grandmother gracefully brings closure to the graveside gathering. She explains that it is the custom of the family for everyone now to share food and conversation and to celebrate life. We all drive in a caravan to an elegant restaurant and are served many courses of colorful and creatively arranged foods. The great-grandmother tells stories, and I see the web of family and friends shimmer with lighthearted laughter.

Goodbyes and gratitudes are expressed. Deeply moved, I drive away listening to a tape of the ecstatic poetry of Rumi.

There is a place where words are born of silence,
A place where the whispers of the heart arise.
There is a place where voices sing your beauty,
A place where every breath
carves your image
in my soul.

Rumi

My body comes to rest as his words lead me home and to spirit.

Gardening Wave—*Andrea Juhan* (psychotherapist)

Flowing: Spring dreams of the garden; the plans, the preparation
Staccato: Late spring work; planting, digging, organizing, implementing
Chaos: High summer when the garden needs everything at once, watering, pruning, fertilizing
Lyrical: Autumn harvest
Stillness: All growth is over, plants rest into compost for next year's garden

Rock 'n' Roll Wave—*Jamie Catto* (rock singer)

I meet up with the guys in the tour bus, all natural and family, *flowing* all the way to the venue. Matty's playing one of his new tunes and everyone's blown away by it. This adds to the growing excitement as we pull up outside the gig.

Doors open. Press and fans yap and push photos of me I've never seen before in my face to sign, sometimes without even any eye contact. I see Max submerged beneath a writhing pile of young teenagers with arms outstretched, black marker pens all around him. Thrilling but not meaningful. The sound check is madness. Equipment smoking. Five hundred strangers running around with scaffolding and strip-plugs, cabling and guitar strings. What have we got ourselves into? "Be careful what you wish for!"

With crackling radio handsets, security guards usher us impersonally toward the back of the stage where we can already hear the overexcited crowd whistling and cheering. As we walk on stage there is an explosion of colored lights, smoke, and sound. I remember nothing for an hour or so as I'm thrown from house to hip-hop, totally absorbed by the rhythms and the screaming (mostly my own). The energy reaches its peak, then dissipates as we leave the crowd with a final moment of gentle gratitude.

After the show the venue empties, leaving cups and leaflets, cigarette butts and silence. We get back on the bus and sleep until we arrive at the next town.

Skiing Wave—*Todd Howard* (ski instructor)

I like to go up to Snowbird early in the morning and exercise my instructor privilege to ride some pre-public trams. With no one else on the mountain I'm free to go wherever I want, as fast as I want. My favorite is when they buff out Regulator. I jump off the lip of the cat track and roll my ski onto edge as I arc my first turn. Four GS turns to the break-over, and then the momentum starts to build. As my edges rip through the corduroy, I make equal turns on both sides of the fall line in sync with my own internal rhythm. When I look back at my tracks, I see the signature of *flowing*.

Snowbird has some of the steepest lift-accesibile terrain anywhere. From the top of Great Scot, you're looking at an eight-foot drop off a cornice into a forty-degree chute. I drop the first turn, make a sharp right and hit a little five-foot floater into the main pocket. My upper body stays quiet; only the lower part works. I breathe out the rhythm in sync with my pole plant. Pole plant, edge check, release—that's *staccato*.

When we get funky snow, I get to see if I can really walk my talk. Three words: breakable wind crust. One second I'm on top of the snow in control, the next I break through and am going way too fast—in a huge trust move, I throw my upper body downhill and thrust my hips out over my feet. Back on top, I keep my edge pressure super light, ready to react to anything. All of my efforts are on balance, no time to think about that last mistake or success. I must be completely present—total *chaos*.

I'm going down the access road and bust ten feet into upper Silver Fox. I land in twenty-seven inches of soft, skied-up crud. I make three short turns to the steep funnel. Two more turns and now I feel I'm reaching terminal velocity. Turn, hit a powder bump and get a big face shot. The next turn is a big fluid arc to the Rock chute. Without checking my speed, I descend into the chute and let my body take over. I'm in the zone, cruising effortlessly and in perfect balance. Spirit is the one skiing this *lyrical* run, but I'm the one with a huge grin on my face.

Once it snowed over eighty inches in five days. The resort hadn't opened for two days because avalanches had crossed the road, closing the canyon. I finally made it up on a blue bird morning. Right before the lifts were to open, another slide crossed the road, closing it till late that afternoon. This left the entire mountain to only a handful of lucky souls. I'd ski along the Traverse and turn hard right off the lip, drop thirty feet, and land in the biggest pile of pillows you can imagine. At the end of a turn I sink under the snow, not to come back up for the next seven turns. No sight, no sound, no breath—only the "White Room." Perfect *stillness*.

Storm Wave—*Kate Engineer* (dancer)

Lying in bed at night in Italy, in a little apartment high on the cliffs, outside my window I can see the place where the blue of the sea meets the blue of the sky. Everything is breathing quietly, the sea breaking on the rocks below in a hypnotic rhythm. I hear the silent pulse of thunder. It escalates until the beat of a gathering storm is tangible. Eventually lightning breaks the sky in big white streaks, illuminating the land for a split second at a time. Flashes come more frequently. The rain pours down; the thunder sounds. All is sound and fury—crashing, elemental, dangerous, exciting—and then it eases, slows down, the rain softens. The dawn is soft and clear. The air sparkles. Everything is new and still and the sun warms away the rain water. The land feels peaceful.

ER Wave—*Jay Kaplan, M.D.*

It's not a bad day in the Emergency Department. A lot of patients, some pretty sick, but no problem I didn't feel comfortable handling. Ambling down the corridors of the ED, I survey the patients and touch base with the nurses caring for them. Abruptly, Katie, the charge nurse, says, "Jay, I need you to see Mr. Garabino on Medical 2—he's got chest pain." There is a sense of tension in the nurse's voice. Is the ease and flow of my day about to be shattered? My heart starts beating faster, I quickly change stride and walk briskly over to the bedside. Mr. Gara-bino is sweating profusely, in obvious distress; he tells me his pain is 10 on a scale of 1 to 10. He looks gray, his eyes and my gut both tell me he's in trouble. The nurses are there, ready . . . O.K., let's start with oxygen, wide open by non-breather mask; two IV's at KVO; aspirin 25 mg orally; a nitroglycerin drip titrated to pain relief. Where's the EKG? I bark. It gets shoved in front of my face. I see he's having a big-time heart attack. What's his blood pressure? "Ninety over sixty," someone calls out. Our actions are perfectly synchronized; we know how to handle this guy.

Suddenly, his eyes roll back and he convulses. A quick look at the cardio monitor—ventricular fibrillation—the rhythmic beating of his heart is lost and his heart is moving like a chaotic bag of worms. Now the methodical, orderly way of doing things is accelerated and we must all act at one time, seemingly chaotic to an outsider, but very grounded. I pound my hand on his chest, the code cart is opened, the defibrillator is charged, the gel pads slapped on his chest, the electrodes applied and—"Everybody off, I'm going to shock him." Wham! His body jerks every which way, but his heart is still fibrillating chaotically. "Give him some lidocaine a hundred mg IV and epi one mg IV. Everybody off." Wham! He jerks again, and this time he responds, his heart shows rhythmic beating, now with occasional irregular, premature beats, skipping along but still pulsing life back into his body. "Another fifty mg of lidocaine and put him on a drip at two mg per minute," I say, smiling at the nurse who receives my order. She smiles back. Mr. Garabino's heart is now beating rhythmically and he's breathing on his own once more. "Blood pressure?" "One-twenty over eighty" is the response. We all breathe a deep sigh of relief and the heavy tension of the previous minutes dissipates. "Okay, now let's give him those other meds—the thrombolytic and the heparin." As Mr. Garabino's eyelids flicker and his eyes dart questioningly around him. "Your heart lost its rhythm for a moment but with a little help it's back in sync; you're going to be OK," I tell him gently and lightly. His eyes are now bright, his color pink, and his skin warm and dry. "What an amazing will to live you have—now is not your time to go," I tell him with a quiet smile as I hold his hand. He knows that he fell into the grave and hopped back out, that he has danced around death and decided that his partner is still life. A few tears well up in the corner of his eye as he focuses on each of us, skipping from one to the other, in thankful communication. We bask in this moment of quiet *stillness,* after one crisis and before the next, realizing that something momentous has taken place and how privileged we are to help a person continue to live.

Fear Wave—*Andrea Juhan*

I'm with my husband and seven-year-old son, Tristan, at a Star Trek convention. After hours of wandering around looking at Star Trek memorabilia we enter the auditorium and take a seat in the balcony to listen to Number One (Riker) speak about the Borg, warp speed, Data, etc.

After a while Tristan has to go to the bathroom. The bathrooms are at the top of the stairs to the right. He's just been there, so I let him go alone this time. I continue to rest and take in Riker. I space out a bit.

I come back to the present with the thought, "Where's Tristan?" He should be back by now, but I figure maybe it hasn't been as long as it seems. I space out a bit more. Then again coming back to the present, I'm thinking he should definitely be back by now and he's not. I feel a low level of anxiety.

I calmly begin to look for him. I go up the stairs around to the men's room, along the hallway. Hmm, no Tristan. Maybe I've missed him and he's back at our seats. I go back to our seats. My husband is there, but not Tristan. My anxiety turns to solid concern.

Up the stairs, back to seat, back to men's room. I can feel the fear taking up more and more space in my body. Moving faster and faster, I no longer can control my mind.

I start freaking out. Where is he? What if he's lost, stolen, kidnapped? Who are all these weird Trekkie people anyway? At this point I'm screaming his name in and out of the auditorium, running in and out of the men's room, in and out of the women's room, up and down the halls. Suddenly I spot him down at the end of the hall by the candy machine.

I am instantly lighter. I run to him with an urgency that knows its goal. Tristan senses my panic, and is confused. He just wants a candy bar. As I take his hand the frantic energy drains out of me and my body quiets.

Bistro Wave—*Martha Clark-Peabody* (artist)

I dress tall
and float thru the dining room
 open the door
 answer the phone
  greet & seat & smile (sweetly) all in one, all at once
   inviting gracious tactful flirtatious
  wearing a servant's heart on my sleeve
 flashing the proprietess/mistress when indeed
  things start to fall apart—
   Sailing out of control
    Too much
    Too little
    Too long of a wait for a table of six
   All wanting & needing & demanding something more
    Bread
    Water
    Attention
   Feed me—serve me—please me—

 steaming plates rushed across the room, wine poured
 and chilled in a bucket too close to the edge of
 the table—watch that glass! This steak is too rare.
 I thought this chicken came with rice. When did you
 open? The music is too loud. The phone is ringing.
 Table 10 wants dessert. Where is your restroom?
   CAN I PLEASE HAVE A FORK
 The well-oiled machine shifts into overdrive
 All needs are met, empty plates are whisked away
  The dance of service winds down into
   A groove of dessert & coffee, sweet with a jolt
   Satisfied exhales of fullness

Companions chatter & laugh playfully fighting over
the candy served at the end of the meal
becoming again the children
   Carefree for a brief moment in time
    Suspended whole.
The door closes
  candles extinguished
   The tables sit silent as I
    Contemplating the clean glasses
     Waiting to be (ful) filled
      once more.

Kid wave—*Vin Marti* (dancer)

For the past six summers I have been leading a workshop in the five rhythms for a group of at-risk inner-city kids in a program called Upward Bound sponsored by the public schools here in Portland.

This past summer I consulted with their teacher and was informed that in school they had been working on the concept of community. I saw this as a great opportunity to show the kids that the five rhythms had practical application "out there" in their world.

After describing the Wave and demonstrating to them what it looks like in my body, I gave them a chance to explore the rhythms, and they did with all the abandonment and curiosity and passion that teenagers can demonstrate when they are turned on. I then gave them each paper and a pencil and took them to a downtown public square where we could witness and record the Wave in action.

The writing they produced was filled with awe and wonder and a sense of intuitive poetry. They witnessed the *flowing* motion of water cascading down bricks. *Staccato* was present in the hackey-sack games going on in the square. Some thought the hand gestures of the Middle Eastern men in conversation looked *chaotic*. The dash of people to catch the next light rail leaving the station struck them as *lyrical*. The quiet and *still* wandering of a pregnant woman through the square hit home for one.

What the kids did next was totally their own doing. A few of them revisited the square with a camera, took pictures of the scene, and, as a commencement exercise, presented to the rest of the school a multimedia showing of the Five Rhythm Wave. Some of the kids danced the rhythms while others read aloud the writings that were recorded that day. Meanwhile, slides of the photographs were shown as a background. I was taught a great deal about my practice that summer.

Egg Wave—*Linda Kahn* (editor)

Flowing—soft-boiled
Staccato—hard-boiled
Chaos—scrambled
Lyrical—sunnyside up
Stillness—poached

Retail Wave—*Janice Hogarth* (marketing executive)

It was the day after Thanksgiving, traditionally the busiest day of the year in retail. I was working in the merchandise department at the Hard Rock Cafe in New York City, selling t-shirts from a narrow counter next to the coat-check window.

On the big day, we had an hour line before we even opened our doors, and it didn't stop for the fifteen hours we were open for business. It was completely frenetic. As many people as possible were allowed inside to stand on the other side of our counter in order to escape the freezing cold temperatures outside, so the room resembled a sardine can. With the Stones, Beatles, and Doors blaring in our ears, everyone had to yell at each other to be heard.

At first, we all flowed together in easy, nurturing, soft movements as the dawn of our day came and went like a smooth Dire Straits album. Our bodies occasionally brushed each other as we folded, arranged, and piled the shirts. Right at lunch hour, our movements became sharper and more focused as the lines grew and people's patience became shorter. Quick and efficient use of our energy was called for, requiring clear *staccato* boundaries. Jagger screamed "Start Me Up" in the background. People were growing hungrier. Our bodies now bumped into each other with more force in our seemingly smaller space.

Just when we thought we couldn't go any faster, breathe any harder, yell any louder, we met *chaos*! Our bodies were flying all over our small space—arms and legs in every direction—as well as t-shirts, hats, and buttons. Customers seemed out of control, throwing their tens, twenties and hundreds at us, spending frantically without thinking twice. (I've noticed *chaos* is a very conducive environment to increasing retail sales levels.) We thought we would all go crazy. But the funny thing is, it didn't happen. We went to the edge, we all lost control, but some of us found that if we stayed in our bodies with our feet on the ground, magic things happened.

And then it all became very light and easy as the Manhattan sky darkened and we entered *lyrical*. The customers suddenly seemed lovely to us. We stopped bumping into each other and our space seemed to expand. We made time to go to the bathroom and fill our bodies with food and drink. We laughed together drunk from the energy of the day.

Then, *stillness*—oh, sweet *stillness*. The music softened. We heard our breathing clearly. Our bodies became quiet. We looked deep into each other's eyes for the first time all day, not yet believing what we had been through.

We broke the Guinness Book of World Records that day for retail sales per square foot, selling more than $86,000 worth of t-shirts and sweatshirts. That's approximately five hundred shirts per hour! That day made a day on the New York Stock Exchange seem like an Enya record.

Meal Wave—*Amber Rose Kaplan* (mom)

I enter the restaurant hungry, join my friends, and order a glass of red wine. I ponder the menu, allowing the different possibilities to flow through my mind and engage my imagination. The waiter meanders to our table and we relay our choices. The soup arrives and I slowly savor its warmth. Next comes the salad with its crunch and crispness. I pitch the crudités and croutons into my mouth and chew and chew until the garden before me disappears. Conversation becomes animated as we each anticipate our individual feasts. The plates are large, so many combinations of tastes to behold! I'm a little overwhelmed, but excited. My dinner fork and knife get moving, dancing their way into *chaos*. I try a bit of this with that, that with this, exchanging bites with dear friends. It's all so good—I'm in ecstasy. I love food! To eat and be aware of the great pleasure we have been given as human beings—Yes, life! Now we're laughing, sharing intimate secrets and stories, hopes and dreams. Not much room left, but just enough for dessert. My spoon dips into the sweetness of a crème brûlée—the simultaneous smoothness and crunch, surprising my senses. It tickles and tiptoes on my tongue, and delicately kisses me with its delicious delights. As the conversation winds down, I sip my café au lait. We pay the bill; some people leave. The meal has come to an end, and in *stillness* I am grateful.

Architectural Wave—*Hans Li* (seeker)

Soul with a hundred thousand bodies
Everything's myself; I talk only of me.
Like a wave I rise in my own body—
Sea and wave the same wild water.

Rumi

Eero Saarinen, TWA Terminal, JFK Airport

Flowing

Staccato!

"Falling Water" Kaufmann House 1936
Frank Lloyd Wright

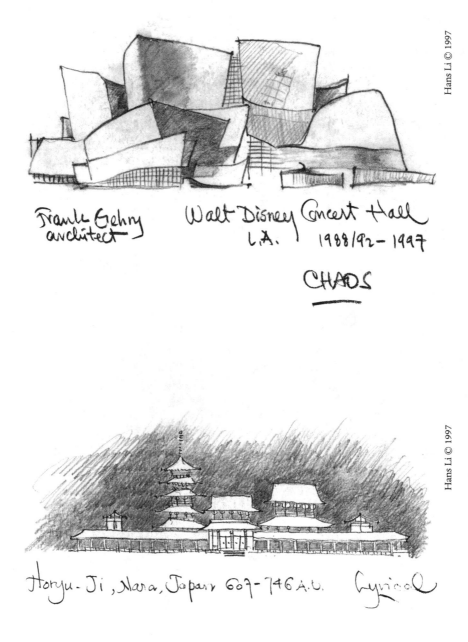

Frank Gehry
architect

Walt Disney Concert Hall
L.A.   1988/92 - 1997

CHAOS

Horyu-Ji, Nara, Japan 607-746 A.D.   Lyrical

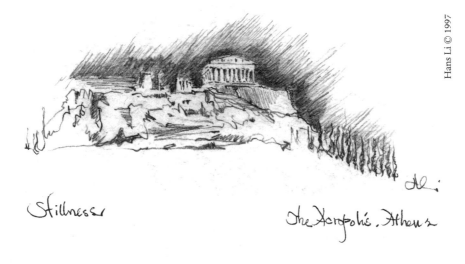

Hans Li © 1997

Stillness   The Acropolis, Athens

Whether on the subway or the ski slope, in the emergency room or the boardroom, practicing the five rhythms helps us become attuned to the underlying patterns in our everyday existence. They teach us that life is energy in motion, freeing us from any fixed notions about people, places, objects, or ideas. Since there is nothing to hold on to, there is nothing to let go.

When things in life seem stuck, my advice is: tread water. Don't identify with the part of you or the situation that is mired in inertia; always identify and go with the part in motion. Keep your head above water and your feet moving, so when the next wave arrives, you'll be ready to ride.

Just as waves are the practice of the water, rhythms are the practice of the body. The body is mostly water, after all. It's our nature to be fluid. The rhythms keep me in touch with this fluidity, with the changing nature of everything except change itself. Only when I recognized the impermanence of my state of being did I sense something truly eternal: a pattern of ceaseless motion with a simple message. It was the same one my nana offerred me years ago in a moment of great pain—this too will pass.

I offer you this as a mantra for whenever you think you are stuck or faced with an intractable problem or an overwhelming grief. Have faith in your process; have faith that the rhythms within you will bear you up and carry you through. All you need to do is surrender and surf the waves.

> *If it's the last dance*
> *Dance backwards.*
>
> *Bo*

TO DO (or NOT TO DO)—Waves

Awareness

All energy moves in one of these five universal rhythms and once you have sorted out which rhythm dominates your life, you have discovered one of the most fundamental things you can know about yourself.

Left to your own devices, how would you move through your day? Imagine you have no obligations, nowhere to go, nothing to do. For some, this might be a scary thought; for others, a luxury. What rhythm do you imagine informing this space? I live in a completely *staccato* and *chaotic* world, but left to my own devices, everything slows down to a very still flow.

Action

Make a list of everybody you know. Beside their name write the rhythm that best describes their energy. Organize your list into posses. The *Flowing* Posse. The *Staccato* Posse. The *Chaos* Posse. The *Lyrical* Posse. The *Still* Posse. If you don't seem to know anybody who fits into one of the rhythms, stop and wonder why.

Do all five rhythms in the following order—*flowing, staccato, chaos, lyrical,* and *stillness*—as a continuous wave to the sound of your own breath. Let the transitions between each rhythm happen, don't make them happen. Do as many waves as you can. When you reach *stillness,* wait for the impulse to *flow* again. When you finish dancing, sit and watch your breath.

Dance the Wave through any of the following:

The Endless Wave, Vol. 1

Bones (songs 2-6)

Trance (songs 4-8)

Initiation (songs 1-5)

EPILOGUE: Tribe

Davida is moving to L.A., so Maryann is throwing her a going-away party at Leon's fifth-floor East Village walkup. The party is off to a languorous start. Tim lies on the couch resting his neck in preparation for the Lollapalooza Tour and purring in Kate's ear. Pierre, a Parisian photographer, shows me his portofolio and we discuss how the five rhythms relate to photography. Lorca squats down next to us and sings us a country love song she wrote. Jonny is massaging Robert's shoulders under the Wandering Jew. Maryann sits on the fire escape smoking cigarettes with Gary, who's looking hot in a tight leopard print shirt—not bad for a computer genius. I meander over and tease him that I'm going to create a five-step program to help all my dancer friends quit smoking. He responds by paraphrasing Rilke—I don't want to kick out my devils because I'm afraid my angels will leave too.

Greg saunters in with some ice-skating friends and begins flirting in his inimitable style. Davida's twin sister, Gabrielle, tells me that although she's taken a few workshops, in this last one she experienced *staccato* for the first time and it was exhilarating. To which Zeet adds, "Lady Bird in Blackness, I am *staccato* and I've yet to take a workshop."

I hand Davida a going-away present. Days before I'd overheard her say that if she had a black dress by my favorite designer, Ghost, she could live happily ever after. I felt like testing this theory and am quite pleased with the way it slinks over her curves and turns her *mistress* on full throttle. L.A. will never be the same.

In the light of the full moon, the silver Deco spire of the Chrysler building is shimmering. I need to dance. I move into the living room, sink into my feet, and surrender to Natasha Atlas singing "Fun Does Not Exist."

Gary stubs out his cigarrette and joins me in the beat. As his body ripples to her undulating voice, I think about the amazing transformation he has undergone. The first time I noticed him in one of my workshops, he was a trembling bundle of nerves as if he had been hit with a triple dose of shy. Now he's dancing like a wild man. Gary epitomizes the spirit of my work: over the past seven years, he has studied with every teacher I've trained, from San Francisco to London, sampling each much as a connoisseur tastes fine wines. He understands that the real teacher is the teaching itself.

Twenty years ago I had a vision while dancing in my living room in San Rafael, overlooking the skyline of the city across the bay. As if struck by a bolt of lightning, I was glued to the floor as a series of images poured through my head. I saw hospitals, schools, churches, theaters, and the rhythms moving through them, like a snake. As I emerged from this trance-state, I knew my work would never be fixed but always fluid; an organism, not an organization; inspirational, not institutional. It would be a marriage of art and healing, restoring life to existing structures rather than creating new ones.

Totally overwhelmed, I called an extraordinary psychic I had met once in the Oklahoma desert. She said: "You've just had a vision, haven't you? Don't be distressed. You won't have to do it alone."

She was right.

Since then, I've gone from being a lone wolf dancing for my own survival to a member of a tribe of dancing maniacs. I've ridden the wave of the five rhythms through *flowing,* when I gave birth to this body of work; through *staccato,* in which I gave it structure. As the work has evolved into its *chaotic* phase, I've been sitting on couches in various parts of the world with a tiny team of tantric terrorists trying to figure it all out. But of course, it can never be figured out or pinned down—it's a body in motion, with its own heart, mind, soul, and spirit.

Every time I dance I shed the skins of separateness and I feel the frequency of tribe. I realize now that tribe is the snake of my vision, which shapeshifted into an international network of people mad about the rhythms. I look out the window at the World Trade Center. The earth doesn't know it has boundaries, doesn't know Peru from California. It's convenient for us to think of it as subdivided—it makes it easier for the anchors on CNN—but in reality it is one. Similarly we may present different aspects of ourselves to different people but we too are one, not just in and of ourselves but one with each other, the earth and the universe. We touch one part of the whole; and another part feels it, there's a resonance, an awareness of being in a bigger picture.

The party is now in full swing. I look up from my dance and see Krishna, surrounded by dancing girls, staring down at me from an antique wall hanging. Inside the sweet embrace of the five rhythms, I have bonded with almost everybody in this room. They are mirrors reflecting back to me all the worlds within the dance. Sometimes they're my students, other times, they're my teachers. But they're always my friends.

And beyond this room the wave continues to ripple out and gather us in. From Susannah and Ya'Acov in London to Kathy and Lori in San Francisco to Martha and Zeet in New Jersey, to Jonny and Angel on the road, to the Maori dancer in New Zealand, to the Zulu priest in South Africa, to the soccer mom in Seattle, we are all part of the Wave, part of the tribe. I now know why I saw a snake in my vision: it's that old serpent again, but this time leading us back into the garden, back to the earth, whole and healed, spirit and flesh reunited.

ENDNOTES

Jewel Mathieson's "Mary Stripped of Duty" and "My Spirit Takes the Wind by Surprise" are from her book, *Silk Tracks Purging Silences from Cells*. Her other poems are works in progress.

All illustrations by: Hans Li © 1997.

Lyrics on p. 139 by Tim Booth from the James' album, *Laid*.

Lyrics on p. 137 by Tim Booth from the album *Booth & The Bad Angel*.

Rumi poetry on p. 2 and p. 208 © translation and re-creation by Andrew Harvey. Rumi poetry on p. 198 translated by J. Star.

ABOUT THE AUTHOR

Gabrielle Roth is an internationally renowned theater director, dance teacher/explorer, and recording artist, and the bestselling author of *Maps to Ecstasy*. Her teaching throughout many areas of culture for the past thirty-five years has included working with thousands of people in settings as diverse as schools, hospitals, corporations, theaters, and growth centers, including Esalen Institute. Gabrielle Roth's work has been featured in *Self, Elle, Mademoiselle, Yoga Journal, Shape,* and many other national publications. Her workshops and retreats have an electric intensity that marries contemporary currents of rock music, modern theater, and poetry to the ancient pulse of shamanism. She lives in New York City.

For further information about the lectures, workshops, trainings, and performance labs of Gabrielle Roth, contact:

THE MOVING CENTER
P.O. Box 2034
Red Bank, NJ 07701
973-642-1979
e-mail: ravenrec@panix.com
http://www.ravenrecording.com

Gabrielle's work can also be explored through the following:

Videos

—*The Wave: Ecstatic Dance for Body & Soul*

The revolutionary moving meditation that first brought Gabrielle's work into the home.

—*I Dance the Body Electric*

Gabrielle in warm and spirited conversation about her unique approach to healing through the creative process and living life as art.

Albums

—*Endless Wave: Vol. 1*

Side One: The soundtrack of Gabrielle's extraordinary video, *The Wave*. Gabrielle guides you through the body parts and Five Rhythms.

Side Two: An unguided tour through the body parts and Five Rhythms set to a hot, new percussion track.

Book

—*Maps to Ecstasy*

Gabrielle's internationally acclaimed book about her work.

Music albums by Gabrielle Roth & The Mirrors:

—*Zone Unknown*

The new one—hot, driving and trancy

—*Stillpoint* (A Compilation)

A collection of Gabrielle's previously-released songs of *stillness*—great for massage, meditation, and yoga

—*Tongues*

A lyrical, upbeat journey through the rhythms

—*Luna* (Nominated for an Indie as Best New Age Album of 1994)

Deep songs that evoke the feminine mysteries—emphasis on *flowing*

—*Trance*

Three warm-up songs lead to the Five Rhythms

—*Waves*

High energy, with a focus on *staccato* and *chaos*

—*Ritual*

Relaxing and inspirational with emphasis on the rhythms of *stillness* and *flowing*

—*Bones*

Hymns to the sacred animal spirits—one warm-up song leads to the Five Rhythms

—*Initiation*

Side One: A journey through the Five Rhythms

Side Two: A musical guide through each of the body parts

—*Totem*

Gabrielle's oldest and most popular; shamanic drumming and trance/dance music

To order, contact:

RAVEN RECORDING
P.O. Box 2034
Red Bank, NJ 07701
1-800-76-RAVEN
1-973-642-1979
e-mail: ravenrec@panix.com
http://www.ravenrecording.com